Basic Pharmacology MCQ

Part I

- **General principles of Pharmacology**
- **Pharmacodynamics**
- **Pharmacokinetics**

Prepared by Dr: Emil Zaki

2026

Copyright and Medical Disclaimer

This book is an educational resource. Pharmacological information changes as evidence, regulatory decisions, and clinical guidelines evolve. Readers must consult official prescribing information, national or local guidelines, and institutional policies before using drug information in clinical practice, The book does not replace professional education, clinical training, or individualized medical judgment.

Drug names are presented primarily by nonproprietary names, Brand names, when mentioned, are used for identification only and do not imply endorsement.

Contents

Chapter 1 - General Principles of Pharmacology

MCQ 1

Pharmacology is best defined as the science that studies:

A. Human anatomy only
B. Drugs and their interactions with living organisms
C. Microorganisms causing disease
D. Surgical treatment of diseases

Answer: B

Explanation: Pharmacology is the scientific study of drugs, including their sources, properties, mechanisms of action, therapeutic uses, adverse effects, and interactions with living organisms.

MCQ 2

Which branch of pharmacology studies the effects of drugs on the body?

A. Pharmacokinetics

B. Pharmacodynamics

C. Toxicology

D. Pharmacogenomics

Answer: B

Explanation: Pharmacodynamics describes what the drug does to the body, including receptor interactions and physiological effects.

MCQ 3

Pharmacokinetics primarily describes:

A. Drug toxicity

B. Drug interactions

C. What the body does to the drug

D. Drug allergy

Answer: C

Explanation: Pharmacokinetics includes drug Absorption, Distribution, Metabolism, and Excretion (ADME).

MCQ 4

Which process is NOT part of pharmacokinetics?

A. Absorption
B. Distribution
C. Receptor binding
D. Elimination

Answer: C

Explanation: Receptor binding is a pharmacodynamic process.

MCQ 5

Which term refers to the official nonproprietary name of a drug?

A. Brand name
B. Chemical name
C. Generic name
D. Trade name

Answer : C

Explanation: The generic name is the standardized nonproprietary name used to identify the active drug ingredient.

MCQ 6

Which of the following is a brand (trade) name?

A. Ibuprofen
B. Amoxicillin
C. Advil®
D. Metformin

Answer: C

Explanation: Advil® is a brand name for ibuprofen.

Clinical Pearl: One generic drug may have multiple brand names.

MCQ 7

Drugs derived from microorganisms include:

A. Digoxin
B. Penicillin
C. Insulin
D. Atropine

Answer: B

Explanation: Penicillin is produced by the fungus Penicillium.

Clinical Pearl: Many antibiotics originate from microorganisms.

MCQ 8

Which route of administration provides the fastest onset of action?

A. Oral
B. Intramuscular
C. Intravenous
D. Subcutaneous

Answer: C

Explanation: Intravenous administration delivers the drug directly into the bloodstream, producing an immediate effect.

Clinical Pearl: IV administration has 100% bioavailability.

MCQ 9

The oral route of drug administration is characterized by:

A. Complete avoidance of first-pass metabolism

B. Immediate drug effect

C. Possible first-pass hepatic metabolism

D. Highest bioavailability

Answer: C

Explanation: Drugs administered orally may undergo first-pass metabolism in the liver before reaching systemic circulation.

MCQ 10

The transdermal route is most suitable for drugs requiring:

A. Immediate emergency treatment

B. Sustained systemic delivery

C. Rapid anesthesia

D. Intravenous access

Answer: B

Explanation: Transdermal patches provide slow, continuous drug absorption over an extended period.

Clinical Pearl: Examples include nicotine and fentanyl patches.

MCQ 11

Drug receptors are usually:

A. Plasma proteins

B. Enzymes

C. Macromolecules that bind drugs and initiate a response

D. Red blood cells

Answer: C

Explanation: Most drug receptors are proteins located on cell membranes or inside cells.

Clinical Pearl: Drug-receptor interaction is the basis of pharmacodynamics.

MCQ 12

An agonist is a drug that:

A. Blocks receptor activation

B. Binds to a receptor and activates it

C. Destroys receptors

D. Prevents drug metabolism

Answer: B

Explanation: Agonists possess both receptor affinity and intrinsic activity.

Clinical Pearl: Full agonists produce the maximum biological response.

MCQ 13

A competitive antagonist:

A. Irreversibly destroys receptors

B. Binds reversibly to the receptor without activating it

C. Produces maximal receptor activation

D. Enhances agonist activity

Answer: B

Explanation: Competitive antagonists compete with agonists for the same receptor and their effects can often be overcome by increasing agonist concentration.

Clinical Pearl: Naloxone is a competitive opioid receptor antagonist.

MCQ 14

The relationship between drug dose and response is described by the:

A. Therapeutic index

B. Dose–response curve

C. Half-life

D. Volume of distribution

Answer: B

Explanation: The dose–response curve illustrates how increasing drug doses affect the magnitude of the response.

Clinical Pearl: Dose–response curves help compare drug potency and efficacy.

MCQ 15

A drug requiring a smaller dose to produce the same effect is considered more:

A. Toxic

B. Selective

C. Potent

D. Effective

Answer: C

Explanation: Potency refers to the amount of drug needed to produce a given effect.

Clinical Pearl: Potency does not necessarily indicate greater clinical benefit.

MCQ 16

The maximum effect a drug can produce is called its:

A. Potency

B. Efficacy

C. Bioavailability

D. Clearance

Answer: B

Explanation: Efficacy (Emax) is the greatest therapeutic response achievable with a drug.

Clinical Pearl: Efficacy is generally more clinically important than potency.

MCQ 17

A drug with a high therapeutic index is generally considered:

A. Less effective

B. More toxic

C. Safer

D. Less potent

Answer: C

Explanation: A high therapeutic index indicates a wide margin between effective and toxic doses.

Clinical Pearl: Penicillins generally have a wider therapeutic index than digoxin.

MCQ 18

Drug selectivity refers to a drug's ability to:

A. Act exclusively on one organ at all doses

B. Preferentially act on one receptor or target over others

C. Avoid metabolism completely

D. Produce the same effect in every patient

Answer: B

Explanation: Selectivity means preferential action on a particular target. Selectivity is relative rather than absolute and may decrease as the dose increases.

Clinical Pearl: No drug is completely specific.

MCQ 19

A patient develops severe anaphylaxis immediately after receiving penicillin. This is an example of which type of adverse drug reaction?

A. Type A (Augmented)

B. Type B (Bizarre)

C. Type C (Chronic)

D. Type E (Withdrawal)

Answer: B

Explanation: Penicillin-induced anaphylaxis is an unpredictable, immune-mediated Type B adverse drug reaction.

Clinical Pearl: Type B reactions are uncommon but may be life-threatening.

MCQ 20

Which statement best describes rational drug use?

A. Prescribing the newest medication available

B. Prescribing multiple drugs for every disease

C. Using medications appropriate to the patient's clinical needs, in the correct dose and duration, at the lowest appropriate cost

D. Prescribing antibiotics for all febrile illnesses

Answer: C

Explanation: The WHO definition of rational medicine use likewise emphasizes appropriate medication, individualized dose, adequate duration, and lowest appropriate cost.

Clinical Pearl: Rational prescribing improves therapeutic outcomes, reduces adverse drug reactions, and helps prevent antimicrobial resistance.

MCQ 21

Which statement best describes bioavailability?

A. The rate of drug metabolism

B. The fraction of an administered dose that reaches the systemic circulation unchanged

C. The duration of drug action

D. The degree of protein binding

Answer: B

Explanation: Bioavailability refers to the proportion of an administered drug that reaches the systemic circulation in an active form. Intravenous drugs have 100% bioavailability.

Clinical Pearl: Oral drugs usually have lower bioavailability because of incomplete absorption and first-pass metabolism.

MCQ 22

Which route of administration completely avoids first-pass hepatic metabolism?

A. Oral

B. Rectal

C. Intravenous

D. Sublingual

Answer: C

Explanation: Intravenous administration delivers the drug directly into the bloodstream, bypassing the liver during initial circulation.

Clinical Pearl: Sublingual drugs also largely avoid first-pass metabolism.

MCQ 23

A patient with severe vomiting requires immediate medication. Which route is most appropriate?

A. Oral

B. Intravenous

C. Topical

D. Rectal

Answer: B

Explanation: Intravenous administration provides rapid drug delivery and is preferred when oral administration is not possible.

Clinical Pearl: IV therapy is commonly used in emergency situations.

MCQ 24

Which receptor type is directly coupled to ion channels?

A. G protein-coupled receptor

B. Enzyme-linked receptor

C. Ligand-gated ion channel

D. Intracellular receptor

Answer: C

Explanation: Ligand-gated ion channels open or close in response to ligand binding, producing rapid cellular responses.

Clinical Pearl: Nicotinic acetylcholine receptors are classic ligand-gated ion channels.

MCQ 25

Intracellular receptors are primarily activated by:

A. Large protein molecules

B. Peptide hormones

C. Lipid-soluble drugs

D. Neurotransmitters

Answer: C

Explanation: Lipid-soluble drugs can cross the cell membrane and bind intracellular receptors.

Clinical Pearl: Steroid hormones act through intracellular receptors.

MCQ 26

A partial agonist produces:

A. No receptor activation

B. Maximum receptor activation

C. Less than the maximum response even when all receptors are occupied

D. Irreversible receptor blockade

Answer: C

Explanation: Partial agonists have affinity for receptors but lower intrinsic activity than full agonists.

Clinical Pearl: Buprenorphine is an example of a partial opioid agonist.

MCQ 27

Which pharmacodynamic parameter represents the maximum achievable drug effect?

A. ED50

B. Half-life

C. Emax

D. Clearance

Answer: C

Explanation: Emax represents the maximum efficacy that a drug can produce.

Clinical Pearl: Increasing the dose beyond Emax does not increase the therapeutic response.

MCQ 28

The ED50 of a drug refers to the dose that:

A. Produces toxicity in 50% of patients

B. Produces the specific therapeutic effect in 50% of the population

C. Is lethal in 50% of animals

D. Is eliminated in 50% of patients

Answer: B

Explanation: ED50 (Median Effective Dose) is the dose producing the desired therapeutic effect in 50% of the population.

MCQ 29

Which drug characteristic is reflected by the position of the dose–response curve along the x-axis?

A. Toxicity

B. Efficacy

C. Potency

D. Selectivity

Answer: C

Explanation: A leftward shift indicates greater potency because less drug is required to achieve the same effect.

MCQ 30

Two drugs produce the same maximum effect, but Drug A requires a lower dose than Drug B. Drug A is:

A. More effective

B. More potent

C. More selective

D. Less safe

Answer: B

Explanation: Drug A is more potent because it achieves the same effect at a lower dose.

Clinical Pearl: Greater potency does not necessarily mean better clinical efficacy.

MCQ 31

Which drug is well known for having a narrow therapeutic index?

A. Amoxicillin

B. Digoxin

C. Paracetamol (Acetaminophen)

D. Cetirizine

Answer: B

Explanation: Digoxin has a narrow therapeutic index, requiring careful dose adjustment and monitoring.

Clinical Pearl: Drugs with narrow therapeutic indices often require therapeutic drug monitoring.

MCQ 32

Which patient is at the greatest risk of developing adverse drug reactions?

A. Healthy young adult

B. Middle-aged athlete

C. Older adult taking multiple medications

D. Healthy teenager

Answer: C

Explanation: Older adults with polypharmacy have increased susceptibility to adverse drug reactions.

Clinical Pearl: Renal impairment and multiple comorbidities further increase the risk.

MCQ 33

Warfarin-induced bleeding is an example of which type of adverse drug reaction?

A. Type A

B. Type B

C. Type D

D. Type E

Answer: A

Explanation: Bleeding from warfarin is predictable, dose dependent, and therefore classified as a Type A ADR.

Clinical Pearl: Type A reactions account for most adverse drug reactions.

MCQ 34

Abrupt discontinuation of long-term corticosteroid therapy may result in:

A. Type A reaction

B. Type B reaction

C. Type E reaction

D. Type F reaction

Answer: C

Explanation: Withdrawal of corticosteroids may cause adrenal insufficiency, a classic Type E reaction.

Clinical Pearl: Corticosteroids should usually be tapered gradually.

MCQ 35

Which of the following best describes pharmacovigilance?

A. Drug manufacturing

B. Monitoring drug prices

C. Detection, assessment, and prevention of adverse drug reactions

D. Drug marketing

Answer: C

Explanation: Pharmacovigilance focuses on identifying and preventing medication-related harm after drugs enter clinical use.

Clinical Pearl: Healthcare professionals should report serious and unexpected adverse drug reactions.

MCQ 36

Which is considered a high-alert medication?

A. Vitamin C

B. Warfarin

C. Calcium carbonate

D. Loratadine

Answer: B

Explanation: Warfarin has a high risk of causing serious harm if used incorrectly.

Clinical Pearl: Other high-alert medications include insulin, heparin, opioids, and chemotherapy agents.

MCQ 37

Medication reconciliation is primarily intended to prevent:

A. Drug manufacturing errors

B. Drug omissions, duplications, and interactions

C. Drug allergies

D. Drug dependence

Answer: B

Explanation: Medication reconciliation compares current medications with new prescriptions during transitions of care.

Clinical Pearl: It should be performed at admission, transfer, and discharge.

MCQ 38

According to the WHO, essential medicines should be:

A. Available only in tertiary hospitals

B. Expensive and highly specialized

C. Available at all times in adequate quantities and affordable

D. Restricted to emergency departments

Answer: C

Explanation: Essential medicines should be continuously available, affordable, and of assured quality.

Clinical Pearl: The WHO Model List of Essential Medicines guides national medicine policies.

MCQ 39

An approved generic drug must have the same:

A. Tablet color only

B. Packaging only

C. Active ingredient, dosage form, strength, and therapeutic effect as the brand-name drug

D. Manufacturer

Answer: C

Explanation: Generic drugs must demonstrate bioequivalence and therapeutic equivalence to the reference product.

Clinical Pearl: Generic substitution improves access to affordable medications.

MCQ 40

Which of the following is the best example of evidence-based pharmacotherapy?

A. Prescribing a drug because a colleague recommends it

B. Choosing therapy based solely on patient preference

C. Selecting medication using current clinical evidence, professional judgment, and patient preferences

D. Always prescribing the newest available medication

Answer: C

Explanation: Evidence-based pharmacotherapy integrates the best available research evidence with clinical expertise and patient values to achieve optimal therapeutic outcomes.

Clinical Pearl: Evidence-based prescribing improves patient safety, treatment effectiveness, and cost-effectiveness.

MCQ 41

A patient receives nitroglycerin sublingually for acute angina. The main advantage of the sublingual route is that it:

A. Produces sustained drug release for several days
B. Avoids first-pass hepatic metabolism and provides rapid absorption
C. Is less expensive than oral administration
D. Prevents all adverse drug reactions

Answer: B

Explanation: Sublingual administration allows rapid absorption through the oral mucosa directly into the systemic circulation, largely bypassing first-pass hepatic metabolism.

Clinical Pearl: Sublingual nitroglycerin typically begins to relieve angina within minutes.

MCQ 42

Which of the following is an example of a pharmacodynamic process?

A. Drug metabolism by the liver
B. Drug excretion by the kidneys
C. Binding of a drug to its receptor
D. Drug absorption from the intestine

Answer: C

Explanation: Pharmacodynamics describes the interaction between drugs and their receptors and the resulting biological effects.

Clinical Pearl: Pharmacodynamics answers the question: What does the drug do to the body?

MCQ 43

Which statement regarding receptor affinity is correct?

A. It describes the maximum effect produced by a drug.
B. It refers to the ability of a drug to bind to its receptor.
C. It measures drug elimination.
D. It determines drug bioavailability.

Answer: B

Explanation: Affinity is the tendency of a drug to bind to its receptor. High-affinity drugs bind more readily.

Clinical Pearl: Affinity and intrinsic activity together determine the pharmacological response.

MCQ 44

Which receptor family is activated through intracellular signaling pathways involving second messengers such as cAMP or IP3?

A. Ligand-gated ion channel

B. G protein-coupled receptor

C. Intracellular receptor

D. Voltage-gated ion channel

Answer: B

Explanation: G protein-coupled receptors activate heterotrimeric G proteins and downstream second-messenger pathways. They mediate many clinically important drug effects.

MCQ 45

A noncompetitive antagonist differs from a competitive antagonist because it:

A. Increases receptor activation
B. Cannot be overcome by increasing the agonist concentration
C. Has greater potency
D. Produces maximal receptor activation

Answer: B

Explanation: Noncompetitive antagonists reduce the maximum response and cannot usually be overcome by increasing agonist concentration.

Clinical Pearl: Noncompetitive antagonists decrease drug efficacy rather than simply shifting the dose-response curve.

MCQ 46

Increasing the dose of a full agonist beyond its maximal efficacy (Emax) will:

A. Increase the maximum response further

B. Decrease potency

C. Produce no additional therapeutic effect but may increase toxicity
D. Convert it into a partial agonist

Answer: C

Explanation: Once Emax is reached, higher doses do not improve efficacy but increase the risk of adverse effects.

Clinical Pearl: "More drug" does not always mean "more benefit."

MCQ 47

Which factor is most likely to reduce the therapeutic index of a drug?

A. Wide margin between effective and toxic doses
B. Narrow difference between effective and toxic doses
C. High bioavailability
D. High receptor selectivity

Answer: B
Explanation: A narrow therapeutic index indicates that toxic effects occur at doses close to therapeutic doses.
Clinical Pearl: Digoxin, lithium, and warfarin require careful monitoring because of their narrow therapeutic indices.

MCQ 48

Drug selectivity is best described as the ability of a drug to:

A. Produce no adverse effects
B. Bind preferentially to a particular receptor or tissue
C. Eliminate rapidly from the body
D. Cross the blood-brain barrier

Answer: B

Explanation: Selective drugs preferentially interact with specific receptors, although complete specificity is rare.

Clinical Pearl: Selectivity often decreases as drug doses increase.

MCQ 49

Which adverse drug reaction is most likely to occur after prolonged drug therapy?

A. Type A

B. Type B

C. Type C

D. Type F

Answer: C

Explanation: Type C (Chronic) reactions are associated with long-term drug use and cumulative exposure.

Clinical Pearl: Long-term corticosteroid therapy causing osteoporosis is a classic example.

MCQ 50

Failure of an oral contraceptive due to rifampicin-induced enzyme induction is classified as:

A. Type A ADR

B. Type B ADR

C. Type E ADR

D. Type F ADR

Answer: D

Explanation: Type F reactions represent failure of therapy, often caused by drug interactions or inadequate dosing.

Clinical Pearl: Rifampicin induces hepatic enzymes and reduces the effectiveness of many medications.

MCQ 51

Which patient characteristic most commonly requires dose adjustment?

A. Brown eye color

B. Renal impairment

C. Left-handedness

D. Blood group O

Answer: B

Explanation: Many drugs are eliminated by the kidneys; impaired renal function can lead to drug accumulation and toxicity.

MCQ 52

Which of the following is an important strategy for preventing medication errors?

A. Using abbreviations whenever possible

B. Confirming patient identity before medication administration

C. Prescribing multiple drugs without review

D. Ignoring patient allergies if the reaction occurred years earlier

Answer: B

Explanation: Correct patient identification is one of the fundamental principles of medication safety.

Clinical Pearl: Always verify at least two patient identifiers before administering medication.

MCQ 53

Which organization introduced the concept of Essential Medicines?

A. American Medical Association (AMA)

B. World Health Organization (WHO)

C. Centers for Disease Control and Prevention (CDC)

D. International Committee of the Red Cross (ICRC)

Answer: B

Explanation: The WHO introduced the Essential Medicines concept in 1977 to improve access to effective, safe, and affordable medicines.

Clinical Pearl: The WHO Model List serves as a guide for national essential medicines lists.

MCQ 54

Which statement regarding generic drugs is TRUE?

A. They contain different active ingredients than brand-name drugs.

B. They must demonstrate bioequivalence to the reference product.

C. They are less effective than brand-name drugs.

D. They are approved without regulatory review.

Answer: B

Explanation: Approved generic drugs must demonstrate bioequivalence and meet the same quality, safety, and efficacy standards as the reference product.

MCQ 55

Which of the following best reflects rational drug prescribing?

A. Prescribing antibiotics for every patient with fever

B. Choosing medications supported by evidence and tailored to the patient's needs

C. Prescribing the most expensive medication available

D. Prescribing medications requested by the patient without assessment

Answer: B

Explanation: Rational prescribing requires selecting evidence-based therapy appropriate for the patient's diagnosis and clinical condition.

Clinical Pearl: Rational prescribing improves outcomes while reducing unnecessary costs.

MCQ 56

The PICO model is primarily used to:

A. Classify adverse drug reactions

B. Formulate answerable clinical questions

C. Measure drug potency

D. Calculate drug half-life

Answer: B

Explanation: PICO stands for Patient (or Problem), Intervention, Comparison, and Outcome.

Clinical Pearl: PICO is widely used in evidence-based medicine to guide literature searches.

MCQ 57

Which type of scientific evidence generally provides the highest level of evidence for therapeutic interventions?

A. Expert opinion

B. Case reports

C. Randomized controlled trials

D. Systematic reviews and meta-analyses

Answer: D

Explanation: Systematic reviews and meta-analyses synthesize results from multiple high-quality studies and generally provide the strongest evidence.

Clinical Pearl: Clinical guidelines are often based on systematic reviews.

MCQ 58

A physician discusses treatment options with a patient, explains benefits and risks, and incorporates the patient's preferences into the final decision. This process is known as:

A. Polypharmacy

B. Shared decision-making

C. Therapeutic duplication

D. Pharmacovigilance

Answer: B

Explanation: Shared decision-making combines clinical evidence with patient values and preferences to select the most appropriate treatment.

Clinical Pearl: Shared decision-making improves adherence and patient satisfaction.

MCQ 59

Which of the following best describes pharmacovigilance?

A. Manufacturing pharmaceutical products

B. Monitoring, detecting, assessing, and preventing adverse drug reactions after drug marketing

C. Measuring drug potency

D. Calculating drug doses

Answer: B

Explanation: Pharmacovigilance focuses on the ongoing monitoring of medication safety throughout a drug's lifecycle.

Clinical Pearl: Reporting suspected adverse drug reactions contributes to safer medication use worldwide.

MCQ 60

A clinician reviews the patient's diagnosis, medical history, kidney function, current medications, allergies, and current clinical guidelines before prescribing therapy. Which principle is being applied?

A. Empirical prescribing

B. Evidence-based and rational pharmacotherapy

C. Polypharmacy

D. Defensive medicine

Answer: B

Explanation: Rational and evidence-based pharmacotherapy integrates clinical evidence with patient-specific factors to select the safest and most effective treatment.

Clinical Pearl: The best prescription is one that is evidence-based, individualized, effective, safe, and acceptable to the patient.

MCQ 61

Which route of drug administration is most appropriate for a patient who is unconscious but has stable circulation?

A. Oral

B. Sublingual

C. Intravenous

D. Topical

Answer: C

Explanation: An unconscious patient cannot safely swallow medications. Intravenous administration provides rapid and reliable drug delivery.

Clinical Pearl: Always assess airway, breathing, and circulation before selecting the route of drug administration.

MCQ 62

A drug that binds to a receptor without activating it and prevents an agonist from binding is called a(n):

A. Full agonist

B. Partial agonist

C. Competitive antagonist

D. Inverse agonist

Answer: C

Explanation: Competitive antagonists bind reversibly to receptors without activating them and compete with agonists for receptor binding.

Clinical Pearl: Increasing the agonist concentration can usually overcome competitive antagonism.

MCQ 63

Which statement regarding efficacy and potency is correct?

A. Potency is more clinically important than efficacy.

B. Efficacy is the maximum response a drug can produce.

C. Potency measures the safety of a drug.

D. Efficacy and potency are always directly proportional.

Answer: B

Explanation: Efficacy refers to the maximum therapeutic effect, whereas potency refers to the amount of drug required to produce a given effect.

Clinical Pearl: When choosing between drugs, efficacy is often more important than potency.

MCQ 64

A patient accidentally receives ten times the prescribed dose of insulin because of a decimal point error. This is an example of:

A. Type B adverse drug reaction

B. Medication error

C. Drug allergy

D. Drug intolerance

Answer: B

Explanation: Incorrect dosing caused by prescribing or administration mistakes is classified as a medication error.

Clinical Pearl: Always avoid trailing zeros (e.g., write 5 mg, not 5.0 mg).

MCQ 65

Which of the following patients is at the greatest risk for medication errors?

A. A healthy young adult taking one medication

B. A hospitalized older adult receiving multiple medications

C. A teenager using topical acne cream

D. An athlete taking vitamin supplements

Answer: B

Explanation: Older hospitalized patients with polypharmacy have a significantly higher risk of medication errors.

MCQ 66

Which statement best describes a high-alert medication?

A. It is available only by prescription.

B. It has a high potential to cause serious patient harm if used incorrectly.

C. It is always expensive.

D. It has no generic equivalent.

Answer: B

Explanation: High-alert medications carry an increased risk of causing significant harm when errors occur.

MCQ 67

Which of the following best illustrates rational drug use?

A. Prescribing antibiotics for every sore throat

B. Prescribing based on pharmaceutical advertisements

C. Choosing evidence-based therapy appropriate for the patient's diagnosis

D. Prescribing multiple drugs without reviewing current medications

Answer: C

Explanation: Rational drug use emphasizes evidence-based, individualized, and cost-effective therapy.

Clinical Pearl: Not every infection requires an antibiotic.

MCQ 68

Which statement regarding essential medicines is TRUE?

A. They are only used in developing countries.

B. They are selected solely because they are inexpensive.

C. They address the priority healthcare needs of the population.

D. They include only antibiotics.

Answer: C

Explanation: Essential medicines are selected based on public health relevance, efficacy, safety, quality, and cost-effectiveness.

Clinical Pearl: Every country may adapt the WHO Model List according to local healthcare needs.

MCQ 69

Which pharmacokinetic process primarily determines how a drug leaves the body?

A. Absorption

B. Distribution

C. Elimination

D. Receptor binding

Answer: C

Explanation: Elimination consists mainly of metabolism and excretion, removing drugs from the body.

Clinical Pearl: Renal and hepatic function strongly influence drug elimination.

MCQ 70

A patient reports taking an over-the-counter herbal supplement while receiving prescription medications. The clinician should primarily consider the possibility of:

A. Increased receptor selectivity

B. Drug interactions

C. Increased bioavailability of all drugs

D. Reduced drug potency only

Answer: B

Explanation: Herbal products may interact with prescription medications by altering drug metabolism or pharmacodynamic effects.

Clinical Pearl: Always ask patients about herbal products and dietary supplements.

MCQ 71

Which of the following is the best example of a narrow therapeutic index drug?

A. Vitamin C

B. Digoxin

C. Amoxicillin

D. Cetirizine

Answer: B

Explanation: Digoxin has a narrow margin between therapeutic and toxic concentrations.

Clinical Pearl: Therapeutic drug monitoring is recommended for several narrow therapeutic index drugs.

MCQ 72

Which enzyme interaction can increase the plasma concentration of a substrate drug?

A. Enzyme induction

B. Enzyme inhibition

C. Increased renal filtration

D. Reduced intestinal absorption

Answer: B

Explanation: Inhibition of a metabolic enzyme can decrease drug metabolism and increase the concentration of its substrate, potentially increasing therapeutic or toxic effects.

MCQ 73

Which healthcare professional is primarily responsible for verifying prescriptions, identifying drug interactions, and counseling patients?

A. Pharmacist

B. Radiologist

C. Physiotherapist

D. Laboratory technologist

Answer: A

Explanation: Pharmacists play a central role in ensuring safe and effective medication use.

Clinical Pearl: Effective collaboration between physicians, pharmacists, and nurses improves medication safety.

MCQ 74

A patient with severe renal impairment is prescribed a drug that is primarily eliminated unchanged by the kidneys. What is the most appropriate general approach?

A. Ignore renal function because the drug is not metabolized by the liver

B. Consider dose or dosing-interval adjustment according to the drug's renal dosing recommendations

C. Automatically double the dose

D. Stop all other medications regardless of indication

Answer: B

Explanation: Reduced renal clearance can cause accumulation of renally eliminated drugs. Dose or interval adjustments should follow the specific drug's pharmacokinetic and clinical guidance.

MCQ 75

A patient develops severe hypotension immediately after receiving the first dose of a medication because of a known pharmacological effect. This reaction is most likely classified as:

A. Type A adverse drug reaction

B. Type B adverse drug reaction

C. Type D adverse drug reaction

D. Type F adverse drug reaction

Answer: A

Explanation: Type A reactions are predictable and related to the known pharmacological action of the drug.

Clinical Pearl: Most adverse drug reactions encountered in clinical practice are Type A.

MCQ 76

Which practice most directly reduces errors during transitions of care?

A. Relying on the patient's memory alone

B. Comparing the patient's medication list with the intended regimen and resolving discrepancies

C. Avoiding documentation of over-the-counter medicines

D. Automatically discontinuing all home medications

Answer: B

Explanation: Medication reconciliation reduces omissions, duplications, dosing discrepancies, and unintended interactions when patients move between care settings.

MCQ 77

A clinician wants to estimate whether a new therapy improves an outcome compared with standard care. Which study design generally provides the strongest direct evidence for a treatment effect?

A. Case report

B. Expert opinion

C. Randomized controlled trial

D. Cross-sectional survey

Answer: C

Explanation: Randomized controlled trials are designed to compare interventions while reducing confounding and are a major source of evidence for causal treatment effects. Systematic reviews may synthesize several trials.

MCQ 78

The use of computerized provider order entry (CPOE) primarily helps reduce:

A. Drug manufacturing costs

B. Prescribing errors

C. Drug metabolism

D. Drug potency

Answer: B

Explanation: CPOE reduces errors caused by illegible handwriting, incomplete prescriptions, and transcription mistakes.

Clinical Pearl: Combining CPOE with clinical decision support systems further improves medication safety.

MCQ 79

Which patient counseling point is MOST important when prescribing a new medication?

A. Explain only the medication cost.

B. Explain the purpose of the medication, how to take it, possible adverse effects, and when to seek medical attention.

C. Tell the patient to double the next dose after any missed dose.

D. Advise the patient to stop the medication if symptoms improve immediately.

Answer: B

Explanation: Clear counseling should cover the medication's purpose, administration, important risks, adherence, and when the patient should seek help. Specific missed-dose instructions should follow the individual drug's labeling.

MCQ 80

A physician prescribes medication after reviewing current clinical guidelines, considering the patient's kidney function, allergies, concurrent medications, treatment goals, and personal preferences. This is the BEST example of:

A. Empirical prescribing

B. Polypharmacy

C. Evidence-based, patient-centered pharmacotherapy

D. Defensive medicine

Answer: C

Explanation: Evidence-based, patient-centered pharmacotherapy combines high-quality scientific evidence with clinical expertise and individual patient factors to optimize treatment outcomes.

Clinical Pearl: Safe prescribing requires balancing efficacy, safety, patient values, and cost-effectiveness while continuously monitoring therapeutic response.

MCQ 81

Which of the following best describes the primary goal of pharmacotherapy?

A. Eliminate all adverse drug reactions

B. Achieve the desired therapeutic effect with minimal toxicity

C. Prescribe the newest available medication

D. Use the highest possible drug dose

Answer: B

Explanation: The goal of pharmacotherapy is to maximize therapeutic benefit while minimizing adverse effects and toxicity.

Clinical Pearl: Always weigh the benefits of treatment against its potential risks.

MCQ 82

A physician prescribes a medication using its generic name rather than its brand name. The main advantage is that it:

A. Guarantees faster drug absorption

B. Reduces medication costs and prescribing errors

C. Increases drug potency

D. Eliminates adverse drug reactions

Answer: B

Explanation: Prescribing by generic name promotes rational prescribing, improves communication, and usually reduces healthcare costs.

Clinical Pearl: Approved generic drugs are therapeutically equivalent to their brand-name counterparts.

MCQ 83

A patient has reduced hepatic function and is receiving a drug extensively metabolized by the liver. What should the prescriber consider?

A. Possible reduction in clearance and the need for individualized dosing

B. Automatic doubling of the dose

C. That liver function cannot affect drug exposure

D. That only renal function matters for all drugs

Answer: A

Explanation: Hepatic dysfunction can reduce metabolism of some drugs and increase exposure. The effect varies by drug and should be assessed using drug-specific guidance.

MCQ 84

Which statement about adverse drug reactions (ADRs) is correct?

A. All ADRs are preventable.

B. Type A reactions are unpredictable.

C. Type A reactions are usually dose dependent and predictable.

D. Type B reactions account for most ADRs.

Answer: C

Explanation: Type A reactions are related to the known pharmacological effects of the drug and are usually predictable and dose dependent.

Clinical Pearl: Approximately 70–80% of ADRs are Type A reactions.

MCQ 85

Which of the following is an example of a medication error?

A. A patient develops a penicillin allergy.

B. A nurse administers medication to the wrong patient.

C. A patient develops nausea after chemotherapy.

D. A patient experiences an expected adverse effect of morphine.

Answer: B

Explanation: Administering medication to the wrong patient is a preventable medication error.

Clinical Pearl: Use at least two patient identifiers before administering medications.

MCQ 86

The WHO Model List of Essential Medicines is primarily intended to:

A. Replace national treatment guidelines.

B. Guide countries in selecting priority medicines.

C. Approve new drugs for marketing.

D. Regulate pharmaceutical prices.

Answer: B

Explanation: The WHO Model List serves as a reference for countries developing their National Essential Medicines Lists.

Clinical Pearl: Essential medicines improve access to safe, effective, and affordable treatment.

MCQ 87

Which statement regarding generic drugs is FALSE?

A. They contain the same active ingredient as the reference drug.

B. They must demonstrate bioequivalence.

C. They usually cost less than brand-name drugs.

D. They require different therapeutic doses than brand-name drugs.

Answer: D

Explanation: Generic drugs contain the same active ingredient and therapeutic dose as the corresponding brand-name product.

Clinical Pearl: Differences in tablet color or shape do not usually affect therapeutic outcomes.

MCQ 88

Which strategy best reduces unnecessary polypharmacy?

A. Adding a medication whenever a new symptom appears

B. Periodically reviewing indications, effectiveness, adverse effects, interactions, and ongoing need for each medication

C. Using only brand-name products

D. Avoiding medication review after discharge

Answer: B

Explanation: Structured medication review can identify medications that are unnecessary, duplicative, ineffective, or causing harm and can support safer deprescribing when appropriate.

MCQ 89

The PICO format is used to:

A. Classify adverse drug reactions.

B. Evaluate medication errors.

C. Develop focused clinical questions for evidence-based practice.

D. Measure therapeutic index.

Answer: C

Explanation: PICO stands for Patient (Problem), Intervention, Comparison, and Outcome and is used to formulate answerable clinical questions.

MCQ 90

Which source is most useful for answering a focused question about the overall effect of an intervention when multiple high-quality randomized trials are available?

A. A single case report

B. An expert anecdote

C. A systematic review and meta-analysis of relevant trials

D. A pharmaceutical advertisement

Answer: C

Explanation: A well-conducted systematic review and meta-analysis can synthesize results across relevant trials and provide an overall estimate of treatment effects, while the quality of the included studies remains important.

MCQ 91

A patient taking five different prescription medications is an example of:

A. Therapeutic duplication

B. Polypharmacy

C. Drug intolerance

D. Pharmacovigilance

Answer: B

Explanation: Polypharmacy is commonly defined as the concurrent use of five or more medications.

Clinical Pearl: Polypharmacy increases the risk of drug interactions and adverse drug reactions.

MCQ 92

Which healthcare professional is primarily responsible for educating patients about the safe use of prescribed medications at the time of dispensing?

A. Pharmacist

B. Radiographer

C. Pathologist

D. Physiotherapist

Answer: A

Explanation: Pharmacists play an important role in medication counseling, identifying interactions, and improving medication adherence.

Clinical Pearl: Effective counseling reduces medication errors and improves therapeutic outcomes.

MCQ 93

A patient is admitted to hospital with a medication list from home. Which process helps verify that the list is complete and accurate and that intended medications are continued, changed, or stopped appropriately?

A. Medication reconciliation

B. Therapeutic duplication

C. Pharmacogenomics

D. First-pass metabolism

Answer: A

Explanation: Medication reconciliation is a structured comparison of medication lists to identify and resolve discrepancies during transitions of care.

MCQ 94

A physician carefully reviews current clinical guidelines before selecting therapy. This practice reflects:

A. Defensive medicine

B. Evidence-based pharmacotherapy

C. Empirical treatment only

D. Therapeutic duplication

Answer: B

Explanation: Evidence-based pharmacotherapy integrates current scientific evidence, clinical expertise, and patient preferences.

Clinical Pearl: Clinical guidelines support—but do not replace—clinical judgment.

MCQ 95

When a patient and clinician discuss the evidence, benefits, risks, alternatives, and the patient's preferences before choosing treatment, the process is called:

A. Shared decision-making

B. Enzyme induction

C. Medication reconciliation

D. Therapeutic drug monitoring

Answer: A

Explanation: Shared decision-making is a collaborative process that incorporates evidence and patient preferences into treatment decisions.

MCQ 96

Which finding is a typical target of post-marketing drug-safety surveillance?

A. Rare adverse reactions that were not apparent in preapproval trials

B. The color of a tablet

C. The manufacturer's advertising budget

D. The patient's preferred pharmacy

Answer: A

Explanation: Post-marketing surveillance can detect rare, delayed, or population-specific adverse effects that may not be apparent in preapproval studies.

MCQ 97

A clinician prescribes the lowest effective dose of a medication to minimize toxicity. Which pharmacological principle is being applied?

A. Irrational prescribing

B. Rational drug use

C. Polypharmacy

D. Therapeutic duplication

Answer: B

Explanation: Using the lowest effective dose reduces the risk of adverse effects while maintaining therapeutic benefit.

Clinical Pearl: "Start low and go slow" is especially important in older adults.

MCQ 98

Which factor should be considered before prescribing any medication?

A. Patient allergies

B. Kidney and liver function

C. Current medications

D. All of the above

Answer: D

Explanation: Safe prescribing requires a comprehensive assessment, including allergies, organ function, concurrent medications, and comorbidities.

Clinical Pearl: A complete medication history helps prevent adverse drug reactions and interactions.

MCQ 99

A patient experiences an unexpected severe allergic reaction after the first dose of a medication despite appropriate prescribing. This event is best classified as:

A. Medication error

B. Type B adverse drug reaction

C. Type A adverse drug reaction

D. Therapeutic failure

Answer: B

Explanation: Type B (Bizarre) reactions are unpredictable, not dose dependent, and often immune-mediated.

Clinical Pearl: Penicillin-induced anaphylaxis is a classic Type B ADR.

MCQ 100

Which statement best summarizes the principles of modern pharmacology?

A. Prescribe the newest medication available regardless of cost.

B. Use multiple medications whenever possible.

C. Select evidence-based, safe, effective, patient-centered therapy while monitoring therapeutic response and adverse effects.

D. Avoid generic medications whenever possible.

Answer: C

Explanation: Modern pharmacology emphasizes rational prescribing, evidence-based medicine, patient safety, individualized therapy, and continuous monitoring to optimize therapeutic outcomes.

References

- Goodman & Gilman's — pharmacologic principles, mechanisms, pharmacodynamics and pharmacokinetics.
- Katzung's Basic & Clinical Pharmacology — especially useful for students and foundational concepts.
- Rang & Dale's Pharmacology — excellent explanations of mechanisms and receptor pharmacology.
- Lippincott Illustrated Reviews: Pharmacology — useful for concise explanations and examination-oriented learning.

Chapter 2 - Pharmacdynamics

MCQ 101

A drug receptor is best defined as:

A. An enzyme responsible for drug metabolism

B. A protein molecule that specifically binds a drug and initiates a biological response

C. A plasma protein that transports drugs in the bloodstream

D. A membrane channel that allows drug excretion

Correct Answer: B

Explanation

Drug receptors are specialized proteins located on the cell membrane, within the cytoplasm, or inside the nucleus. They bind drugs or endogenous ligands and initiate cellular responses.

A is incorrect because enzymes metabolize drugs.

C is incorrect because plasma proteins transport drugs but are not receptors.

D is incorrect because excretion is performed by organs such as the kidneys and liver.

Clinical Pearl: Most clinically useful drugs act by interacting with specific receptors.

MCQ 102

Which of the following is the most common type of drug receptor?

A. DNA polymerase

B. G protein-coupled receptor (GPCR)

C. Hemoglobin

D. Albumin

Correct Answer: B

Explanation

G protein-coupled receptors (GPCRs) represent the largest family of drug receptors and mediate the actions of many hormones, neurotransmitters, and therapeutic agents.

- A is an enzyme.
- C transports oxygen.
- D is the major plasma protein responsible for drug binding.

Clinical Pearl: Approximately one-third of currently prescribed drugs act through GPCRs.

MCQ 103

A drug that binds to a receptor and produces a biological response is called:

A. Antagonist

B. Partial inhibitor

C. Agonist

D. Chelating agent

Correct Answer: C

Explanation

An agonist binds to a receptor and activates it, producing a biological effect.

- A blocks receptor activation.
- B is not a standard pharmacological term in this context.
- D binds metals rather than receptors.

MCQ 104

Drug receptors are most commonly composed of:

A. Lipids

B. Carbohydrates

C. Proteins

D. DNA

Correct Answer: C

Explanation

Most drug receptors are proteins with highly specific binding sites for endogenous ligands and drugs.

- Lipids and carbohydrates are structural components but rarely function as drug receptors.
- DNA is the target of only selected drugs.

MCQ 105

Which receptor type directly regulates gene transcription after activation?

A. Ligand-gated ion channel

B. G protein-coupled receptor

C. Nuclear receptor

D. Voltage-gated sodium channel

Correct Answer: C

Explanation

Nuclear receptors are intracellular receptors that regulate gene expression after binding lipid-soluble ligands such as steroid hormones.

Examples include receptors for:

- Cortisol
- Aldosterone
- Estrogen
- Thyroid hormone
- Vitamin D

MCQ 106

Which receptor type mediates the rapid effects of acetylcholine at the neuromuscular junction?

A. Nuclear receptor

B. G protein-coupled receptor

C. Ligand-gated ion channel

D. Tyrosine kinase receptor

Correct Answer: C

Explanation

Nicotinic acetylcholine receptors are ligand-gated ion channels that rapidly open sodium channels after acetylcholine binding.

This results in skeletal muscle contraction within milliseconds.

MCQ 107

The interaction between a drug and its receptor is primarily based on:

A. Covalent binding only

B. Non-specific lipid dissolution

C. Complementary molecular shape and chemical forces

D. Active transport across the membrane

Correct Answer: C

Explanation

Drug-receptor binding depends on molecular complementarity and weak reversible forces, including:

- Hydrogen bonds
- Ionic bonds
- Hydrophobic interactions
- Van der Waals forces

Most therapeutic drugs bind reversibly.

MCQ 108

Affinity refers to:

A. The maximum response a drug can produce

B. The ability of a drug to bind to its receptor

C. The rate of drug metabolism

D. Drug elimination by the kidneys

Correct Answer: B

Explanation

Affinity describes how strongly a drug binds to its receptor.

High-affinity drugs bind receptors effectively even at low concentrations.

Affinity should not be confused with efficacy.

MCQ 109

Intrinsic activity (efficacy) is best defined as:

A. The ability of a drug to bind plasma proteins

B. The ability of a drug to activate a receptor after binding

C. Drug absorption from the gastrointestinal tract

D. Drug metabolism by CYP450 enzymes

Correct Answer: B

Explanation

Intrinsic activity (also called efficacy) is the ability of a drug to activate its receptor and produce a biological response after binding.

- Full agonists have maximal intrinsic activity.
- Partial agonists have reduced intrinsic activity.
- Antagonists have no intrinsic activity.

MCQ 110

Which of the following statements regarding receptors is TRUE?

A. All receptors are located on the cell membrane.

B. Receptors are static structures that never change.

C. Receptors may undergo upregulation or downregulation in response to chronic drug exposure.

D. Every drug exerts its effects through a receptor.

Correct Answer: C

Explanation

Receptors are dynamic structures that adapt to prolonged stimulation or blockade.

- Chronic agonist exposure often causes downregulation.
- Chronic antagonist exposure often causes upregulation.
- A is incorrect because many receptors are intracellular.
- B is incorrect because receptor regulation is a key pharmacological principle.
- D is incorrect because some drugs act through non-receptor mechanisms (e.g., antacids, osmotic diuretics).

MCQ 111

The primary mechanism by which most drugs produce their therapeutic effects is by:

A. Increasing body temperature

B. Binding to specific receptors and modifying cellular function

C. Destroying all microorganisms directly

D. Increasing blood volume

Correct Answer: B

Explanation

Most drugs exert their effects by interacting with specific receptors, enzymes, ion channels, or transport proteins, thereby altering normal cellular function.

- A is unrelated to the mechanism of action of most drugs.
- C applies only to certain antimicrobial agents.
- D is not the general mechanism of drug action.

Clinical Pearl: Drugs modify existing physiological processes—they do not create new biological functions.

MCQ 112

Which receptor type produces the fastest pharmacological response?

A. Nuclear receptor

B. Ligand-gated ion channel

C. G protein-coupled receptor (GPCR)

D. Intracellular steroid receptor

Correct Answer: B

Explanation

Ligand-gated ion channels open within milliseconds after agonist binding, producing rapid changes in membrane potential.

Examples include:

- Nicotinic acetylcholine receptor
- GABA-A receptor
- A and D act by regulating gene transcription, requiring hours to days.
- C acts through second messengers and is slower than ion channels.

MCQ 113

Activation of G protein-coupled receptors (GPCRs) typically leads to:

A. Direct DNA replication

B. Formation of intracellular second messengers

C. Immediate protein synthesis only

D. Permanent receptor destruction

Correct Answer: B

Explanation

GPCR activation stimulates intracellular second messenger systems such as:

- cAMP
- IP_3
- DAG
- Calcium

These signaling pathways regulate numerous physiological responses.

MCQ 114

Insulin exerts its pharmacological effects primarily through which receptor type?

A. Ligand-gated ion channel

B. Nuclear receptor

C. Tyrosine kinase receptor

D. G protein-coupled receptor

Correct Answer: C

Explanation

The insulin receptor is a receptor tyrosine kinase. Binding of insulin activates intracellular phosphorylation pathways that regulate glucose uptake, metabolism, and cell growth.

MCQ 115

Steroid hormones such as cortisol produce their effects by:

A. Blocking sodium channels

B. Binding intracellular receptors and altering gene transcription

C. Opening calcium channels immediately

D. Activating membrane transport pumps only

Correct Answer: B

Explanation

Steroid hormones are lipid-soluble and diffuse across cell membranes to bind intracellular (cytoplasmic or nuclear) receptors, leading to altered gene transcription and protein synthesis.

Their onset of action is slower but their effects are longer-lasting.

MCQ 116

Which of the following drugs acts primarily by inhibiting an enzyme?

A. Aspirin

B. Morphine

C. Salbutamol (Albuterol)

D. Atropine

Correct Answer: A

Explanation

Aspirin irreversibly inhibits cyclooxygenase (COX-1 and COX-2), reducing prostaglandin and thromboxane synthesis.

- Morphine activates opioid receptors.

- Salbutamol stimulates β_2-adrenergic receptors.
- Atropine blocks muscarinic receptors.

Clinical Pearl: Not all drugs act through receptors; many act by inhibiting enzymes.

MCQ 117

Which of the following is an example of a drug acting on an ion channel?

A. Lidocaine blocking voltage-gated sodium channels

B. Warfarin inhibiting vitamin K recycling

C. Digoxin inhibiting Na^+/K^+-ATPase

D. Omeprazole inhibiting the proton pump

Correct Answer: A

Explanation

Lidocaine blocks voltage-gated sodium channels, preventing nerve impulse conduction and producing local anesthesia.

- B, C, and D act on enzymes or membrane pumps rather than ion channels.

MCQ 118

Which statement best describes second messengers?

A. They transport drugs in plasma.

B. They transmit intracellular signals after receptor activation.

C. They metabolize drugs in the liver.

D. They eliminate drugs through the kidneys.

Correct Answer: B

Explanation

Second messengers relay signals from activated cell-surface receptors to intracellular targets.

Common second messengers include:

- cAMP
- cGMP
- IP_3
- DAG
- Calcium ions (Ca^{2+})

MCQ 119

Digoxin produces its therapeutic effect by inhibiting:

A. Cyclooxygenase (COX)

B. Na^{+}/K^{+}-ATPase pump

C. Acetylcholinesterase

D. Monoamine oxidase (MAO)

Correct Answer: B

Explanation

Digoxin inhibits the sodium-potassium ATPase pump, increasing intracellular calcium in cardiac muscle and enhancing myocardial contractility.

This mechanism is useful in selected patients with heart failure and atrial fibrillation.

MCQ 120

Which of the following statements regarding mechanisms of drug action is TRUE?

A. Every drug acts through a receptor.

B. Drugs create entirely new physiological functions.

C. Drugs modify existing physiological or pathological processes.

D. All drugs act by changing gene transcription.

Correct Answer: C

Explanation

Drugs modify existing physiological or pathological processes by interacting with receptors, enzymes, ion channels, transporters, or nucleic acids.

- A is incorrect because some drugs act through non-receptor mechanisms (e.g., osmotic diuretics, antacids).
- B is incorrect because drugs do not create new biological functions.
- D is incorrect because only selected drugs (e.g., steroid hormones) alter gene transcription directly.

MCQ 121

An agonist is best defined as a drug that:

A. Binds to a receptor without producing a response

B. Binds to a receptor and activates it to produce a biological effect

C. Prevents drug metabolism

D. Inhibits drug absorption

Correct Answer: B

Explanation

An agonist binds to a receptor and activates it, producing a biological response. Agonists possess both affinity (ability to bind) and intrinsic activity (efficacy) (ability to activate the receptor).

- A describes an antagonist.
- C and D are unrelated to receptor activation.

Clinical Pearl: Agonists mimic the action of endogenous substances such as hormones and neurotransmitters.

MCQ 122

Which of the following drugs is a full agonist at the μ-opioid receptor?

A. Naloxone

B. Buprenorphine

C. Morphine

D. Atropine

Correct Answer: C

Explanation

Morphine is a full μ-opioid receptor agonist, producing maximal analgesic effects.

- Naloxone is an opioid antagonist.
- Buprenorphine is a partial agonist.
- Atropine is a muscarinic receptor antagonist.

MCQ 123

A partial agonist is a drug that:

A. Produces no receptor activation

B. Produces a maximal response equal to a full agonist

C. Produces a submaximal response even when all receptors are occupied

D. Permanently blocks receptors

Correct Answer: C

Explanation

Partial agonists bind to receptors but produce less than the maximum possible response, even when all receptors are occupied.

Example:

- Buprenorphine at μ-opioid receptors.

MCQ 124

An antagonist differs from an agonist because it:

A. Has affinity but no intrinsic activity

B. Has intrinsic activity but no affinity

C. Produces maximal receptor activation

D. Always binds irreversibly

Correct Answer: A

Explanation

Naloxone is a competitive opioid receptor antagonist that reversibly displaces opioid agonists from their receptors.

- Phenoxybenzamine is an irreversible α-adrenergic antagonist.
- Aspirin inhibits cyclooxygenase.
- Ketamine is a noncompetitive NMDA receptor antagonist.

Clinical Pearl: Naloxone is the drug of choice for opioid overdose.

MCQ 125

Which of the following is a competitive antagonist?

A. Phenoxybenzamine

B. Naloxone

C. Aspirin

D. Ketamine

Correct Answer: B

Explanation

Naloxone is a competitive opioid receptor antagonist that reversibly displaces opioid agonists from their receptors.

- Phenoxybenzamine is an irreversible α-adrenergic antagonist.
- Aspirin inhibits cyclooxygenase.
- Ketamine is a noncompetitive NMDA receptor antagonist.
- Clinical Pearl: Naloxone is the drug of choice for opioid overdose.

MCQ 126

Increasing the concentration of an agonist can overcome the effects of which type of antagonist?

A. Noncompetitive antagonist

B. Competitive antagonist

C. Chemical antagonist

D. Physiological antagonist

Correct Answer: B

Explanation

Competitive antagonists bind reversibly to the same receptor site as the agonist.

Increasing agonist concentration can displace the antagonist and restore the response.

MCQ 127

Which statement regarding noncompetitive antagonists is TRUE?

A. They produce a rightward shift without changing Emax.

B. Their effects are completely overcome by increasing agonist concentration.

C. They reduce the maximum response (Emax).

D. They always increase drug potency.

Correct Answer: C

Explanation

Noncompetitive antagonists reduce the maximum achievable response (Emax) because receptor function cannot be fully restored by increasing agonist concentration.

MCQ 128

Buprenorphine is best classified as a:

A. Full agonist

B. Partial agonist

C. Competitive antagonist

D. Irreversible antagonist

Correct Answer: B

Explanation

Buprenorphine is a partial μ-opioid receptor agonist.

It provides analgesia with a ceiling effect on respiratory depression, making it useful in opioid dependence treatment.

MCQ 129

Which of the following drugs is a muscarinic receptor antagonist?

A. Salbutamol (Albuterol)

B. Atropine

C. Pilocarpine

D. Dopamine

Correct Answer: B

Explanation

Atropine competitively blocks muscarinic acetylcholine receptors.

Clinical uses include:

- Symptomatic bradycardia
- Organophosphate poisoning
- Preoperative reduction of secretions

- Pilocarpine is a muscarinic agonist.
- Salbutamol is a β_2-adrenergic agonist.
- Dopamine is a dopamine receptor agonist.

MCQ 130

Which of the following statements about agonists and antagonists is TRUE?

A. Antagonists have greater intrinsic activity than agonists.

B. Full agonists produce the maximum possible receptor response.

C. Partial agonists have no affinity for receptors.

D. Competitive antagonists decrease Emax.

Correct Answer: B

Explanation

Full agonists produce the maximum biological response by fully activating receptors.

- A is incorrect because antagonists have no intrinsic activity.
- C is incorrect because partial agonists have both affinity and intrinsic activity.
- D is incorrect because competitive antagonists do not reduce Emax; they increase EC50 and shift the dose-response curve to the right.

MCQ 131

A dose–response relationship describes the relationship between:

A. Drug cost and therapeutic benefit

B. Drug dose and the magnitude of the biological response

C. Drug absorption and elimination

D. Drug metabolism and excretion

Correct Answer: B

Explanation

A dose–response relationship illustrates how the magnitude of a drug's effect changes as the dose or concentration increases. It is fundamental for determining drug potency, efficacy, and optimal dosing.

A is unrelated to pharmacodynamics.

C and D describe pharmacokinetics rather than dose–response relationships.

Clinical Pearl: Dose–response curves help clinicians determine safe and effective drug doses.

MCQ 132

Which parameter represents the maximum effect that a drug can produce?

A. EC50

B. ED50

C. Emax

D. Therapeutic Index

Correct Answer: C

Explanation

Emax is the maximum response that can be achieved with a drug, regardless of further dose increases.

- EC50 is the concentration producing 50% of the maximal effect.
- ED50 is the median effective dose in quantal studies.
- Therapeutic Index measures drug safety.

MCQ 133

The EC50 of a drug is defined as:

A. The dose producing toxic effects in 50% of individuals

B. The concentration producing 50% of the maximal response

C. The concentration causing death in 50% of individuals

D. The dose producing the maximum response

Correct Answer: B

Explanation

EC50 (Half-Maximal Effective Concentration) is the concentration of a drug that produces 50% of its maximum effect.

A lower EC50 indicates greater potency.

MCQ 134

A drug with a lower EC50 compared with another drug is considered:

A. Less potent

B. More toxic

C. More potent

D. Less efficacious

Correct Answer: C

Explanation

A lower EC50 means that less drug is required to produce a given effect, indicating greater potency.

Potency should not be confused with efficacy.

MCQ 135

Increasing the dose of a full agonist beyond its Emax will:

A. Produce a greater therapeutic response

B. Increase receptor affinity

C. Not increase the maximal therapeutic effect but may increase adverse effects

D. Convert it into a partial agonist

Correct Answer: C

Explanation

Once Emax is reached, further dose increases do not improve therapeutic benefit but increase the likelihood of adverse drug reactions.

MCQ 136

A graded dose–response curve is primarily used to evaluate:

A. The proportion of individuals responding to a drug

B. The relationship between dose and response in a single individual or isolated tissue

C. Drug elimination half-life

D. Drug bioavailability

Correct Answer: B

Explanation

Graded dose–response curves measure the magnitude of response as drug concentration increases in an individual or tissue preparation.

They are commonly used to determine:

- Potency
- Efficacy
- EC50
- Emax

MCQ 137

A quantal dose–response curve measures:

A. Continuous changes in blood pressure

B. The percentage of individuals who exhibit a specified response at different doses

C. Plasma drug concentration over time

D. Drug distribution volume

Correct Answer: B

Explanation

Quantal dose–response curves evaluate all-or-none responses in a population.

Examples include:

- Sleep achieved
- Pain relief
- Mortality
- Seizure prevention

These curves are useful for determining ED50, TD50, and LD50.

MCQ 138

Which statement regarding graded and quantal dose–response curves is TRUE?

A. Both measure identical pharmacological responses.

B. Graded curves evaluate individuals, whereas quantal curves evaluate populations.

C. Quantal curves determine receptor affinity.

D. Graded curves measure only toxic responses.

Correct Answer: B

Explanation

- Graded dose–response curves measure the magnitude of response in individuals or isolated tissues.
- Quantal dose–response curves measure the proportion of a population achieving a predefined response.

MCQ 139

Which parameter is commonly determined from a quantal dose–response curve?

A. EC50

B. Emax

C. ED50

D. Volume of distribution

Correct Answer: C

Explanation

ED50 (Median Effective Dose) is derived from quantal dose–response curves and represents the dose that produces the desired effect in 50% of the population.

MCQ 140

Which of the following statements regarding dose–response relationships is TRUE?

A. Potency is determined by Emax.

B. Emax reflects the maximum therapeutic response achievable by a drug.

C. EC50 measures drug safety.

D. Increasing the dose always increases the therapeutic response.

Correct Answer: B

Explanation

Emax represents the maximum effect that a drug can produce.

- Potency is measured by EC50.
- Drug safety is evaluated using the Therapeutic Index, not EC50.
- Increasing the dose beyond Emax increases toxicity rather than therapeutic benefit.

MCQ 141

Drug potency is best defined as:

A. The maximum effect a drug can produce

B. The amount of drug required to produce a specified effect

C. The safety of a drug at therapeutic doses

D. The duration of drug action

Correct Answer: B

Explanation

Potency refers to the dose or concentration of a drug required to produce a given effect. A more potent drug achieves the same response at a lower dose than a less potent drug.

- A describes efficacy.
- C relates to the therapeutic index.
- D refers to the duration of action.

Clinical Pearl: Potency determines how much drug is needed, not how effective the drug ultimately is.

MCQ 142

Drug efficacy is best defined as:

A. The affinity of a drug for its receptor

B. The maximum therapeutic effect that a drug can produce

C. The rate of drug elimination

D. The percentage of drug bound to plasma proteins

Correct Answer: B

Explanation

Efficacy refers to the maximum response (Emax) achievable with a drug, regardless of dose.

- A refers to affinity.
- C concerns pharmacokinetics.
- D relates to drug distribution.

MCQ 143

A drug with a lower EC50 than another drug is:

A. Less potent

B. More efficacious

C. More potent

D. Less safe

Correct Answer: C

Explanation

A lower EC50 indicates that a smaller concentration of the drug is needed to produce 50% of the maximal response, indicating greater potency.

EC50 does not directly measure efficacy or safety.

MCQ 144

Which parameter is used to measure drug efficacy?

A. EC50

B. ED50

C. Emax

D. Therapeutic Index

Correct Answer: C

Explanation

Emax represents the maximum effect that a drug can produce and is therefore the measure of drug efficacy.

MCQ 145

Two drugs produce the same maximum effect, but Drug A requires one-tenth the dose of Drug B.

Which statement is correct?

A. Drug A has greater efficacy.

B. Drug A has greater potency.

C. Drug B has greater potency.

D. Drug B has greater efficacy.

Correct Answer: B

Explanation

Since both drugs produce the same maximum response, they have equal efficacy.

Drug A is more potent because it requires a much lower dose to achieve the same effect.

MCQ 146

Which statement regarding potency and efficacy is TRUE?

A. Potency is more clinically important than efficacy.

B. A highly potent drug always has greater efficacy.

C. Efficacy is generally more important clinically because it determines the maximum therapeutic benefit.

D. Potency and efficacy always increase together.

Correct Answer: C

Explanation

Although potency influences dose selection, efficacy is generally more important because it determines the greatest therapeutic effect a drug can achieve.

A drug may be highly potent but have lower efficacy than another drug.

MCQ 147

Which of the following drugs has lower efficacy than morphine at the μ-opioid receptor?

A. Fentanyl

B. Buprenorphine

C. Hydromorphone

D. Methadone

Correct Answer: B. Buprenorphine.

Explanation

Buprenorphine is a partial μ-opioid receptor agonist and therefore has lower maximal efficacy than full agonists such as morphine, fentanyl, hydromorphone, and methadone.

MCQ 148

A leftward shift of a graded dose–response curve indicates:

A. Decreased efficacy

B. Increased toxicity

C. Increased potency

D. Reduced receptor affinity

Correct Answer: C

Explanation

A leftward shift means that a lower concentration of drug is required to produce the same response, indicating greater potency.

The maximum response (Emax) remains unchanged if efficacy is unchanged.

MCQ 149

Which of the following statements is TRUE regarding a full agonist?

A. It has no intrinsic activity.

B. It produces only a partial response even when all receptors are occupied.

C. It produces the maximum possible response after receptor activation.

D. It always has lower potency than a partial agonist.

Correct Answer: C

Explanation

A full agonist has maximal intrinsic activity and can produce the highest possible biological response when sufficient receptors are occupied.

- A describes an antagonist.
- B describes a partial agonist.
- D is incorrect because potency and efficacy are independent properties.

MCQ 150

Which statement regarding potency and efficacy is CORRECT?

A. Potency describes the maximum therapeutic effect of a drug.

B. Efficacy describes the dose required to produce a response.

C. A more potent drug is always the better therapeutic choice.

D. Potency relates to EC50, whereas efficacy relates to Emax.

Correct Answer: D

Explanation

Potency is measured by EC50, while efficacy is measured by Emax.

Clinical drug selection is usually based more on efficacy, safety, patient factors, and adverse-effect profile than on potency alone.

- A and B incorrectly interchange the definitions.
- C is incorrect because greater potency does not necessarily make a drug clinically superior.

MCQ 151

Receptor downregulation is best defined as:

A. An increase in receptor number after prolonged antagonist therapy

B. A decrease in receptor number or responsiveness following prolonged agonist stimulation

C. Permanent destruction of all receptors

D. Increased drug metabolism by the liver

Correct Answer: B

Explanation

Downregulation occurs when continuous or excessive stimulation by an agonist decreases the number or sensitivity of receptors, reducing the cellular response to the drug.

- A describes upregulation.
- C is incorrect because receptors are continually synthesized and degraded.
- D relates to pharmacokinetics rather than receptor regulation.

Clinical Pearl: Chronic stimulation with agonists often results in diminished responsiveness due to receptor downregulation.

MCQ 152

Receptor upregulation most commonly occurs after:

A. Prolonged agonist stimulation

B. Long-term receptor blockade with antagonists

C. Acute drug overdose

D. Increased drug metabolism

Correct Answer: B

Explanation

Long-term use of receptor antagonists may increase receptor number or sensitivity, a phenomenon known as upregulation.

MCQ 153

Abrupt discontinuation of long-term β-blocker therapy may cause:

A. Bradycardia only

B. Rebound tachycardia and hypertension due to receptor upregulation

C. Immediate receptor destruction

D. Complete loss of β-receptors

Correct Answer: B

Explanation

Chronic β-blocker use causes β-receptor upregulation. Abrupt withdrawal exposes these receptors to circulating catecholamines, leading to rebound sympathetic stimulation.

Possible consequences include:

- Tachycardia
- Hypertension
- Angina
- Myocardial infarction in susceptible patients

MCQ 154

Which of the following best describes desensitization?

A. Increased receptor synthesis after antagonist therapy

B. Reduced receptor responsiveness despite continued agonist exposure

C. Permanent receptor blockade

D. Increased drug absorption

Correct Answer: B

Desensitization is a reduction in receptor responsiveness after repeated or continuous agonist stimulation.

Mechanisms include:

- Receptor phosphorylation

- G-protein uncoupling
- Receptor internalization

MCQ 155

A patient using an inhaled β_2-agonist several times daily notices that the medication becomes progressively less effective.

The most likely explanation is:

A. Receptor upregulation

B. Downregulation of β_2-adrenergic receptors

C. Increased drug absorption

D. Increased receptor synthesis

Correct Answer: B

Explanation

Frequent use of β_2-agonists such as salbutamol (albuterol) may produce β_2-receptor downregulation, decreasing bronchodilator responsiveness.

MCQ 156

Which phenomenon develops within minutes to hours after repeated drug administration?

A. Drug tolerance

B. Tachyphylaxis

C. Upregulation

D. Cross-tolerance

Correct Answer: B

Explanation

Tachyphylaxis is a rapidly developing reduction in drug response caused by receptor desensitization or depletion of endogenous mediators.

Example:

- Ephedrine
- Oxymetazoline nasal spray

MCQ 157

Long-term opioid therapy commonly results in:

A. Receptor upregulation and hypersensitivity

B. Receptor downregulation and drug tolerance

C. Increased receptor synthesis only

D. Complete receptor blockade

Correct Answer: B

Explanation

Chronic opioid exposure causes receptor adaptation, including downregulation and desensitization, leading to tolerance and the need for higher doses to achieve the same analgesic effect.

MCQ 158

Which of the following is the best example of receptor upregulation?

A. Long-term salbutamol therapy

B. Chronic morphine use

C. Long-term propranolol therapy

D. Repeated administration of ephedrine

Correct Answer: C

Explanation

Long-term treatment with propranolol, a β-adrenergic antagonist, increases β-receptor number and sensitivity.

Abrupt withdrawal may produce rebound cardiovascular effects.

MCQ 159

Which statement regarding receptor regulation is TRUE?

A. Receptors remain unchanged throughout life.

B. Downregulation increases receptor sensitivity.

C. Receptor regulation helps maintain physiological homeostasis.

D. Upregulation occurs only in liver disease.

Correct Answer: C

Explanation

Receptor regulation is an adaptive mechanism that maintains homeostasis during prolonged stimulation or inhibition.

It influences therapeutic response, tolerance, and rebound phenomena.

MCQ 160

Which statement regarding receptor regulation is CORRECT?

A. Downregulation usually follows prolonged agonist stimulation.

B. Upregulation occurs after chronic agonist therapy.

C. Desensitization permanently destroys receptors.

D. Receptor regulation has no clinical significance.

Correct Answer: A

Explanation

Prolonged stimulation by agonists commonly leads to downregulation, reducing receptor number or responsiveness.

- Upregulation typically follows chronic antagonist therapy.
- Desensitization is usually reversible.
- Receptor regulation has major clinical implications in chronic drug therapy.

MCQ 161

A competitive antagonist is a drug that:

A. Irreversibly binds to the receptor and permanently blocks it

B. Binds reversibly to the same receptor site as the agonist without activating it

C. Activates the receptor while blocking agonist binding

D. Binds to an intracellular receptor and increases gene transcription

Correct Answer: B

Explanation

A competitive antagonist binds reversibly to the same (orthosteric) receptor site as the agonist, preventing agonist binding without activating the receptor.

- A describes an irreversible antagonist.
- C is incorrect because antagonists have no intrinsic activity.
- D describes activation of nuclear receptors.

Clinical Pearl: The effects of competitive antagonists can usually be overcome by increasing the concentration of the agonist.

MCQ 162

Which of the following is a classic example of a competitive antagonist?

A. Phenoxybenzamine

B. Naloxone

C. Aspirin

D. Digoxin

Correct Answer: B

Explanation

Naloxone is a competitive antagonist at μ-opioid receptors and rapidly reverses opioid-induced respiratory depression.

- Phenoxybenzamine is an irreversible α-adrenergic antagonist.
- Aspirin inhibits cyclooxygenase (COX).
- Digoxin inhibits the Na^+/K^+-ATPase pump.

MCQ 163

The effect of a competitive antagonist can usually be overcome by:

A. Decreasing the agonist dose

B. Increasing the agonist concentration

C. Blocking receptor synthesis

D. Inhibiting drug metabolism

Correct Answer: B

Explanation

Because competitive antagonists bind reversibly, increasing the agonist concentration allows the agonist to compete successfully for receptor occupancy.

MCQ 164

A competitive antagonist typically produces which change in a graded dose–response curve?

A. Decreases Emax only

B. Shifts the curve to the right without changing Emax

C. Shifts the curve to the left

D. Increases both potency and efficacy

Correct Answer: B

Explanation

Competitive antagonism decreases potency (higher EC50), causing a rightward shift of the dose–response curve, while Emax remains unchanged.

MCQ 165

A noncompetitive antagonist differs from a competitive antagonist because it:

A. Can always be displaced by increasing agonist concentration

B. Reduces the maximum response (Emax) of the agonist

C. Has intrinsic activity equal to a full agonist

D. Increases receptor sensitivity

Correct Answer: B

Explanation

Noncompetitive antagonists either bind irreversibly to the agonist-binding site or bind to an allosteric site, reducing the maximum response (Emax). Their effect cannot be fully overcome by increasing agonist concentration.

MCQ 166

Which of the following is a classic example of an irreversible (noncompetitive) antagonist?

A. Naloxone

B. Atropine

C. Phenoxybenzamine

D. Propranolol

Correct Answer: C

Explanation

Phenoxybenzamine irreversibly blocks α_1- and α_2-adrenergic receptors by forming covalent bonds, producing prolonged receptor blockade.

Clinical use:

- Pheochromocytoma

MCQ 167

Which statement regarding noncompetitive antagonism is TRUE?

A. Increasing agonist concentration completely restores the maximal response.

B. EC50 decreases while Emax increases.

C. Emax decreases because functional receptors are unavailable.

D. It always shifts the dose–response curve to the left.

Correct Answer: C

Explanation

Noncompetitive antagonists reduce the number or function of available receptors, thereby lowering Emax. Increasing agonist concentration cannot fully restore the maximal effect.

MCQ 168

A patient receives naloxone after an opioid overdose. Naloxone reverses the opioid effects because it:

A. Irreversibly destroys opioid receptors

B. Competitively displaces opioid agonists from the receptor

C. Stimulates opioid receptor synthesis

D. Inhibits opioid metabolism

Correct Answer: B

Explanation

Naloxone has a higher affinity for μ-opioid receptors than most opioid agonists and competitively displaces them, rapidly reversing respiratory depression.

MCQ 169

Which of the following statements correctly compares competitive and noncompetitive antagonists?

A. Both decrease Emax to the same extent.

B. Competitive antagonists decrease potency, whereas noncompetitive antagonists decrease efficacy.

C. Competitive antagonists permanently bind receptors.

D. Noncompetitive antagonists always increase receptor sensitivity.

Correct Answer: B

Explanation

- Competitive antagonists reduce potency by increasing EC50 but do not reduce Emax.
- Noncompetitive antagonists reduce efficacy by lowering Emax.

MCQ 170

Which statement regarding antagonists is CORRECT?

A. Competitive antagonists reduce Emax.

B. Noncompetitive antagonists can always be overcome by increasing agonist concentration.

C. Competitive antagonists have affinity but no intrinsic activity.

D. Noncompetitive antagonists increase agonist potency.

Correct Answer: C

Explanation

Competitive antagonists bind receptors (affinity) but do not activate them (no intrinsic activity).

- A is incorrect because competitive antagonists do not reduce Emax.
- B is incorrect because noncompetitive antagonism cannot be overcome by increasing agonist concentration.
- D is incorrect because noncompetitive antagonists decrease efficacy rather than increasing potency.

MCQ 171

Drug tolerance is best defined as:

A. An allergic reaction occurring after the first dose of a drug

B. A gradual decrease in drug response requiring larger doses to achieve the same therapeutic effect

C. Complete absence of drug effect after one dose

D. A predictable adverse drug reaction

Correct Answer: B

Explanation

Drug tolerance is a reduction in the response to a drug after repeated administration, resulting in the need for higher doses to produce the same effect.

Mechanisms include:

- Receptor downregulation
- Receptor desensitization
- Increased drug metabolism
- Physiological adaptation
- A describes hypersensitivity.
- C is incorrect because tolerance develops gradually.
- D refers to an adverse drug reaction.

Clinical Pearl: Tolerance commonly develops during long-term therapy with opioids, nitrates, and benzodiazepines.

MCQ 172

Tachyphylaxis is best described as:

A. A gradual decrease in drug response over several months

B. A rapidly developing decrease in drug response after repeated administration over a short period

C. Increased drug absorption after chronic use

D. Permanent receptor destruction

Correct Answer: B

Explanation

Tachyphylaxis is a rapidly developing reduction in drug response, occurring within minutes or hours after repeated dosing.

Mechanisms include:

- Receptor desensitization
- Depletion of endogenous mediators

MCQ 173

Which of the following drugs commonly produces tolerance during long-term therapy?

A. Morphine

B. Penicillin

C. Omeprazole

D. Metformin

Correct Answer: A

Explanation

Chronic opioid therapy leads to tolerance, requiring progressively larger doses for the same analgesic effect.

Tolerance develops to:

- Analgesia
- Euphoria
- Respiratory depression

Tolerance develops poorly, if at all, to:

- Constipation
- Miosis

MCQ 174

Which drug is classically associated with tachyphylaxis?

A. Ephedrine

B. Digoxin

C. Aspirin

D. Warfarin

Correct Answer: A

Explanation

Repeated administration of ephedrine, an indirectly acting sympathomimetic, rapidly depletes norepinephrine stores, producing tachyphylaxis.

Other examples include:

- Oxymetazoline nasal spray
- Tyramine

MCQ 175

The major difference between tolerance and tachyphylaxis is:

A. Tolerance develops rapidly, whereas tachyphylaxis develops over weeks.

B. Tachyphylaxis develops rapidly, whereas tolerance usually develops gradually over days to weeks.

C. Both develop at identical rates.

D. Tachyphylaxis occurs only with antibiotics.

Correct Answer: B

Explanation

- Tolerance develops gradually with repeated exposure.
- Tachyphylaxis develops rapidly after closely repeated doses.

MCQ 176

A patient using nitroglycerin continuously develops reduced anti-anginal efficacy after several days.This phenomenon is best described as:

A. Drug allergy

B. Drug tolerance

C. Idiosyncratic reaction

D. Hypersensitivity

Correct Answer: B

Explanation

Continuous nitrate therapy commonly causes tolerance, reducing anti-anginal efficacy.

Prevention:

- Daily nitrate-free interval of approximately 10–12 hours.

MCQ 177

Which mechanism contributes to drug tolerance?

A. Increased receptor sensitivity only

B. Receptor downregulation and desensitization

C. Complete receptor destruction after one dose

D. Reduced hepatic metabolism in all patients

Correct Answer: B

Explanation

Mechanisms of tolerance include:

- Receptor downregulation
- Receptor desensitization
- Increased drug metabolism

MCQ 178

Which statement regarding tachyphylaxis is TRUE?

A. It is prevented by increasing every drug dose indefinitely.

B. It commonly results from depletion of endogenous neurotransmitter stores.

C. It occurs only with opioid analgesics.

D. It always requires months to develop.

Correct Answer: B

Explanation

Indirectly acting sympathomimetics such as ephedrine depend on endogenous norepinephrine stores.

Repeated dosing rapidly depletes these stores, resulting in tachyphylaxis.

MCQ 179

A patient receiving long-term opioid therapy requires progressively larger doses to maintain adequate pain control.

This is an example of:

A. Drug allergy

B. Drug tolerance

C. Tachyphylaxis

D. Idiosyncrasy

Correct Answer: B

Explanation

Tolerance develops during prolonged opioid therapy because of receptor adaptation and other pharmacodynamic changes.

Dose escalation should always be balanced against the increased risk of adverse effects.

MCQ 180

Which statement regarding drug tolerance and tachyphylaxis is CORRECT?

A. Both terms describe identical pharmacological phenomena.

B. Tolerance develops over time, whereas tachyphylaxis develops rapidly.

C. Tachyphylaxis always results from enzyme induction.

D. Tolerance is caused only by receptor upregulation.

Correct Answer: B

Explanation

Tolerance and tachyphylaxis both reduce drug responsiveness but differ primarily in the speed of onset.

- Tolerance develops gradually over days, weeks, or months.
- Tachyphylaxis develops within minutes or hours.

MCQ 181

A drug interaction is best defined as:

A. A predictable adverse drug reaction occurring at high doses

B. The alteration of the effect of one drug by another drug, food, herbal product, or disease

C. Drug metabolism occurring in the liver only

D. Drug excretion through the kidneys

Correct Answer: B

Explanation

A drug interaction occurs when the pharmacological effect, efficacy, or toxicity of one drug is altered by another drug, food, herbal medicine, dietary supplement, or disease state.

- A describes only one possible consequence of a drug interaction.
- C and D describe pharmacokinetic processes rather than drug interactions.

Clinical Pearl: Drug interactions are a major cause of preventable adverse drug events and hospital admissions.

MCQ 182

Which type of drug interaction occurs when two intravenous medications are physically incompatible after being mixed?

A. Pharmacodynamic interaction

B. Pharmaceutical interaction

C. Food–drug interaction

D. Herb–drug interaction

Correct Answer: B

Explanation

Pharmaceutical interactions occur before administration, usually because of physical or chemical incompatibility between medications.

Examples include:

- Drug precipitation
- Color change
- Loss of drug activity
- Incompatibility

MCQ 183

Which of the following is a classic CYP450 enzyme inducer?

A. Clarithromycin

B. Ketoconazole

C. Rifampicin

D. Erythromycin

Correct Answer: C

Explanation

Rifampicin is a potent inducer of CYP450 enzymes, especially CYP3A4, increasing drug metabolism and reducing plasma concentrations of many medications.

Examples affected include:

- Oral contraceptives
- Warfarin
- Corticosteroids
- Antiretroviral drugs

MCQ 184

Which of the following is a well-known CYP450 enzyme inhibitor?

A. Phenytoin

B. Phenobarbital

C. Carbamazepine

D. Ketoconazole

Correct Answer: D

Explanation

Ketoconazole strongly inhibits CYP3A4, reducing the metabolism of many drugs and increasing the risk of toxicity.

Other important inhibitors include:

- Clarithromycin
- Erythromycin
- Fluconazole
- Ritonavir
- Verapamil
- Amiodarone

MCQ 185

A patient taking warfarin begins treatment with trimethoprim–sulfamethoxazole and subsequently develops bleeding.

The most likely explanation is:

A. Increased renal excretion of warfarin

B. Inhibition of warfarin metabolism leading to increased anticoagulant effect

C. Reduced absorption of warfarin

D. Enhanced vitamin K synthesis

Correct Answer: B

Explanation

Trimethoprim–sulfamethoxazole inhibits the metabolism of warfarin, increasing the INR and significantly raising the risk of bleeding.

Patients receiving this combination require close INR monitoring and possible warfarin dose adjustment.

MCQ 186

Grapefruit juice increases the plasma concentration of several drugs because it:

A. Induces hepatic CYP2D6 enzymes

B. Inhibits intestinal CYP3A4 enzymes

C. Accelerates gastric emptying

D. Increases renal drug excretion

Correct Answer: B

Explanation

Grapefruit juice inhibits intestinal CYP3A4, increasing the bioavailability and plasma concentrations of several medications.

Examples include:

- Simvastatin
- Atorvastatin
- Felodipine
- Amlodipine

MCQ 187

Which food may reduce the anticoagulant effect of warfarin?

A. Apples

B. Bananas

C. Spinach

D. Rice

Correct Answer: C

Explanation

Spinach is rich in vitamin K, which antagonizes the effects of warfarin.

Patients should maintain a consistent intake of vitamin K-rich foods rather than avoiding them completely.

MCQ 188

Which herbal product is a potent CYP3A4 inducer that may reduce the effectiveness of oral contraceptives and warfarin?

A. Ginkgo biloba

B. Ginseng

C. St. John's Wort

D. Echinacea

Correct Answer: C

Explanation

St. John's Wort induces CYP3A4, increasing the metabolism of many drugs and reducing their therapeutic effects.

Clinically important interactions occur with:

- Oral contraceptives
- Warfarin
- Cyclosporine
- HIV medications

MCQ 189

Which of the following drugs has a narrow therapeutic index and therefore requires close monitoring for drug interactions?

A. Amoxicillin

B. Digoxin

C. Paracetamol (Acetaminophen)

D. Cetirizine

Correct Answer: B

Explanation

Digoxin has a narrow therapeutic index; small increases in plasma concentration can cause serious toxicity.

Other drugs with narrow therapeutic indices include:

- Warfarin
- Lithium
- Phenytoin
- Theophylline
- Tacrolimus

MCQ 190

Which statement regarding drug interactions is CORRECT?

A. All drug interactions are harmful.

B. Competitive drug interactions occur only during drug absorption.

C. Drug interactions may be beneficial, harmful, or clinically insignificant.

D. Food has no clinically significant effect on drug therapy.

Correct Answer: C

Explanation

Drug interactions are not always harmful.

Some are intentionally beneficial, such as:

- Levodopa + Carbidopa
- Trimethoprim + Sulfamethoxazole

Others may be harmful or have little clinical significance depending on the drugs involved and the patient.

MCQ 191

A patient receives naloxone after an opioid overdose and rapidly regains consciousness. Naloxone acts as a:

A. Full agonist

B. Partial agonist

C. Competitive antagonist

D. Noncompetitive antagonist

Correct Answer: C

Explanation

Naloxone is a competitive antagonist at μ-opioid receptors. It reversibly binds to opioid receptors and displaces opioid agonists such as morphine and heroin.

- A and B are incorrect because naloxone has no intrinsic activity.
- D is incorrect because naloxone binds reversibly, not irreversibly.

Clinical Pearl: Naloxone is the drug of choice for reversing opioid-induced respiratory depression.

MCQ 192

Which receptor type is responsible for the actions of insulin?

A. G protein-coupled receptor (GPCR)

B. Ligand-gated ion channel

C. Tyrosine kinase receptor

D. Nuclear receptor

Correct Answer: C

Explanation

Insulin binds to a receptor tyrosine kinase, activating intracellular phosphorylation pathways that regulate glucose uptake, metabolism, and cell growth.

MCQ 193

A drug produces the same maximum effect as Drug X but requires only one-fourth of the dose.

Compared with Drug X, this drug is:

A. More efficacious

B. More potent

C. Less potent

D. Less efficacious

Correct Answer: B

Explanation

Because both drugs achieve the same Emax, they have equal efficacy.

The drug requiring the lower dose is more potent because it has a lower EC50.

MCQ 194

Long-term treatment with a β_2-adrenergic agonist may result in:

A. Receptor upregulation

B. Receptor downregulation

C. Increased receptor synthesis only

D. Permanent receptor destruction

Correct Answer: B

Explanation

Prolonged stimulation of β_2-receptors causes receptor downregulation and desensitization, reducing the bronchodilator response over time.

MCQ 195

Which statement regarding competitive antagonists is TRUE?

A. They reduce Emax.

B. Their effects cannot be overcome by increasing agonist concentration.

C. They shift the dose–response curve to the right without changing Emax.

D. They permanently inactivate receptors.

Correct Answer: C

Explanation

Competitive antagonists increase EC50 (decreasing potency) and shift the dose–response curve to the right while preserving Emax.

MCQ 196

Which of the following is the best example of tachyphylaxis?

A. Reduced response to morphine after several months of therapy

B. Rapid loss of response to repeated doses of ephedrine within hours

C. Bleeding after warfarin overdose

D. Anaphylaxis after penicillin administration

Correct Answer: B

Explanation

Tachyphylaxis develops rapidly, often because of depletion of endogenous neurotransmitter stores or rapid receptor desensitization.

Ephedrine is the classic example.

MCQ 197

A patient taking warfarin is prescribed rifampicin. What is the most likely outcome?

A. Increased anticoagulant effect and bleeding

B. Reduced warfarin metabolism

C. Reduced anticoagulant effect due to enzyme induction

D. No clinically significant interaction

Correct Answer: C

Explanation

Rifampicin is a potent CYP450 inducer that accelerates warfarin metabolism, reducing its plasma concentration and anticoagulant effect.

Patients require close INR monitoring and dose adjustment.

MCQ 198

Which receptor type produces the slowest onset of drug action?

A. Ligand-gated ion channel

B. G protein-coupled receptor

C. Tyrosine kinase receptor

D. Nuclear receptor

Correct Answer: D

Explanation

Nuclear receptors regulate gene transcription and protein synthesis. Because these processes require time, the onset of action is measured in hours to days.

Examples include receptors for:

- Cortisol
- Thyroid hormone
- Estrogen
- Vitamin D

MCQ 199

Which statement correctly distinguishes potency from efficacy?

A. Potency refers to Emax, whereas efficacy refers to EC50.

B. Potency indicates the dose needed to produce an effect, whereas efficacy indicates the maximum response achievable.

C. Potency and efficacy always increase together.

D. Potency is more clinically important than efficacy in every situation.

Correct Answer: B

Explanation

- Potency is determined by EC50 and reflects the amount of drug required to produce a specified response.
- Efficacy is determined by Emax and reflects the maximum therapeutic effect a drug can achieve.

MCQ 200

Which of the following statements regarding pharmacodynamics is CORRECT?

A. Pharmacodynamics studies what the body does to the drug.

B. Pharmacodynamics focuses on drug absorption, metabolism, and excretion.

C. Pharmacodynamics studies what the drug does to the body, including receptor interactions and biological responses.

D. Pharmacodynamics is synonymous with pharmacokinetics.

Correct Answer: C

Explanation

Pharmacodynamics is the study of what the drug does to the body, including:

- Drug–receptor interactions
- Mechanisms of drug action
- Dose–response relationships
- Potency
- Efficacy
- Therapeutic and adverse effects

References

- Brunton, L. L., Hilal-Dandan, R., & Knollmann, B. C., eds. Goodman & Gilman's The Pharmacological Basis of Therapeutics. McGraw Hill.
- Katzung, B. G., & Vanderah, T. W. Basic & Clinical Pharmacology. McGraw Hill.
- Ritter, J. M., Flower, R. J., Henderson, G., Loke, Y. K., MacEwan, D., & Rang, H. P. Rang & Dale's Pharmacology. Elsevier.
- Whalen, K. Lippincott Illustrated Reviews: Pharmacology. Wolters Kluwer.
- Katzung, B. G. Trevor's Basic & Clinical Pharmacology Review. McGraw Hill.
- Neal, M. J. Medical Pharmacology at a Glance. Wiley-Blackwell.
- World Health Organization. WHO Model List of Essential Medicines. World Health Organization.
- U.S. Food and Drug Administration. Drugs@FDA: FDA-Approved Drugs. U.S. Food and Drug Administration.
- Goodman & Gilman's – The Pharmacological Basis of Therapeutics
- Rang & Dale's Pharmacology

Chapter 3 - Pharmacokinetics

MCQ 201

What does pharmacokinetics primarily describe?

A. What the drug does to the body

B. What the body does to the drug

C. The therapeutic effects of a drug

D. The toxic effects of a drug

Correct answer: B.

Explanation: Pharmacokinetics describes the movement of drugs through the body, including absorption, distribution, metabolism, and excretion (ADME).

MCQ 202

Which of the following is NOT one of the four major pharmacokinetic processes?

A. Absorption

B. Distribution

C. Receptor activation

D. Excretion

Correct answer: C. Receptor activation

Explanation: Absorption, distribution, metabolism, and excretion are the major pharmacokinetic processes. Receptor activation is primarily pharmacodynamics.

MCQ 203

The fraction of an administered dose that reaches the systemic circulation unchanged is called:

A. Clearance

B. Bioavailability

C. Volume of distribution

D. Extraction ratio

Correct answer: B. Bioavailability

Explanation: Bioavailability (F) is the fraction of the administered dose that reaches systemic circulation as unchanged drug.

MCQ 204

Which route of administration generally has a bioavailability of 100%?

A. Oral
B. Subcutaneous
C. Intravenous
D. Intramuscular

Correct answer: C. Intravenous

Explanation: Intravenous administration delivers the drug directly into the systemic circulation, giving complete bioavailability.

MCQ 205

A major disadvantage of oral administration is:

A. Complete bioavailability
B. First-pass metabolism
C. Immediate onset in all cases
D. Inability to produce systemic effects

Correct answer: B. First-pass metabolism

Explanation: Drugs absorbed from the gastrointestinal tract may undergo significant hepatic metabolism before reaching systemic circulation.

MCQ 206

The first-pass effect occurs primarily in the:

A. Kidney
B. Lung
C. Liver
D. Spleen

Correct answer: C. Liver

Explanation: Drugs absorbed from the gastrointestinal tract enter the portal circulation and may be extensively metabolized in the liver before reaching systemic circulation.

MCQ 207

Which route can largely avoid hepatic first-pass metabolism?

A. Oral

B. Sublingual

C. Enteral feeding tube

D. Oral solution

Correct answer: B. Sublingual

Explanation: Sublingual absorption drains directly into systemic circulation, largely bypassing the portal circulation and first-pass hepatic metabolism.

MCQ 208

Which factor generally increases the rate of dissolution of a solid oral drug?

A. Smaller particle size

B. Larger particle size

C. Reduced surface area

D. Increased crystallinity in all cases

Correct answer: A. Smaller particle size

Explanation: Smaller particles have greater surface area, which generally increases dissolution and may enhance absorption.

MCQ 209

Passive diffusion of drugs across biological membranes generally depends on:

A. ATP consumption

B. A concentration gradient

C. A specific receptor

D. Antibody binding

Correct answer: B. A concentration gradient

Explanation: Passive diffusion occurs down a concentration gradient and does not require cellular energy.

MCQ 210

Which property generally facilitates passive diffusion across lipid membranes?

A. High lipid solubility
B. Permanent ionization
C. Large molecular size
D. Strong plasma protein binding

Correct answer: A. High lipid solubility

Explanation: Lipid-soluble, nonionized drugs generally cross biological membranes more readily by passive diffusion.

MCQ 211

Weak acids are generally more nonionized in:

A. Acidic environments
B. Alkaline environments
D. All environments equally
C. Neutral environments only

Correct answer: A. Acidic environments

Explanation: Weak acids are more likely to remain nonionized in acidic environments, facilitating membrane diffusion.

MCQ 212

Weak bases are generally more nonionized in:

A. Acidic environments
B. Alkaline environments
C. Strongly acidic urine
D. All environments equally

Correct answer: B. Alkaline environments

Explanation: Weak bases become less ionized as the environment becomes more alkaline.

MCQ 213

Ion trapping occurs because:

A. Ionized molecules cross membranes more readily

B. Drugs become permanently lipid soluble

C. Ionized molecules cross lipid membranes poorly

D. All drugs become protein bound

Correct answer: C. Ionized molecules cross lipid membranes poorly

Explanation: A drug can accumulate on the side of a membrane where it becomes ionized and therefore less able to diffuse back.

MCQ 214

Which route provides relatively rapid systemic absorption without requiring gastrointestinal absorption?

A. Oral
B. Sublingual
C. Intravenous
D. Enteral

Correct answer: C. Intravenous

Explanation: IV administration places the drug directly into the bloodstream.

MCQ 215

Intramuscular absorption can be influenced by:

A. Local blood flow
B. Drug formulation
C. Injection site
D. All of the above

Correct answer: D. All of the above

Explanation: Blood flow, formulation, and injection site can all affect the rate of IM drug absorption.

MCQ 216

Bioavailability of an orally administered drug is reduced by:

A. Complete absorption without metabolism
B. First-pass metabolism
C. Intravenous administration
D. Direct arterial injection

Correct answer: B. First-pass metabolism

Explanation: Presystemic metabolism reduces the amount of unchanged drug reaching systemic circulation.

MCQ 217

A drug has an oral bioavailability of 50%. If 200 mg is administered orally, approximately how much reaches systemic circulation unchanged?

A. 25 mg
B. 50 mg
C. 100 mg
D. 200 mg

Correct answer: C. 100 mg

Explanation: Amount reaching systemic circulation = dose × F = 200 × 0.5 = 100 mg.

MCQ 218

A drug with high first-pass metabolism will usually have:

A. Increased oral bioavailability
B. Reduced oral bioavailability
C. 100% oral bioavailability
D. No hepatic metabolism

Correct answer: B. Reduced oral bioavailability

Explanation: Extensive first-pass metabolism can substantially reduce the systemic availability of an orally administered drug.

MCQ 219

Distribution refers to:

A. Chemical modification of a drug
B. Movement of drug between body compartments
C. Removal of drug through urine
D. Binding of drug to receptors only

Correct answer: B. Movement of drug between body compartments

Explanation: Distribution describes the reversible movement of drug from blood into tissues and body fluids.

MCQ 220

Which organ receives a particularly high blood flow and therefore may receive drugs rapidly?

A. Adipose tissue

B. Bone

C. Brain

D. Tendon

Correct answer: C. Brain

Explanation: Highly perfused organs such as the brain, liver, and kidneys generally receive drugs rapidly after systemic administration.

MCQ 221

Plasma protein binding generally produces:

A. An increase in free drug concentration

B. A reservoir of bound drug

C. Immediate elimination of the drug

D. Complete drug metabolism

Correct answer: B. A reservoir of bound drug

Explanation: Protein-bound drug is generally not immediately available for diffusion, metabolism, or filtration and may serve as a reversible reservoir.

MCQ 222

The pharmacologically active fraction of many drugs is primarily the:

A. Protein-bound fraction

B. Free fraction

C. Metabolized fraction

D. Excreted fraction

Correct answer: B. Free fraction

Explanation: Unbound drug is generally available to cross membranes, interact with targets, and undergo elimination.

MCQ 223

Albumin predominantly binds:

A. Many acidic drugs
B. Only carbohydrates
C. Only electrolytes
D. All basic drugs exclusively

Correct answer: A. Many acidic drugs

Explanation: Albumin is an important plasma protein for binding many acidic and neutral drugs.

MCQ 224

A drug that is highly protein bound may be affected by:

A. Changes in plasma protein concentration
B. Drug displacement interactions
C. Changes in binding affinity
D. All of the above

Correct answer: D. All of the above

Explanation: Changes in protein concentration or binding interactions can alter the free concentration of highly protein-bound drugs.

MCQ 225

Volume of distribution (Vd) is best described as:

A. The actual anatomical volume occupied by a drug
B. A theoretical volume relating amount of drug in the body to plasma concentration
C. The volume of urine produced
D. The volume of blood filtered by the kidney

Correct answer: B. A theoretical volume relating amount of drug in the body to plasma concentration

Explanation: Vd is a proportionality constant: Vd = amount of drug in the body / plasma drug concentration.

MCQ 226

A very large Vd generally suggests that the drug:

A. Remains primarily in plasma
B. Is extensively distributed into tissues
C. Is completely excreted
D. Cannot cross membranes

Correct answer: B. Is extensively distributed into tissues

Explanation: A large Vd indicates relatively low plasma concentration compared with the amount of drug in the body, often because substantial drug has entered tissues.

MCQ 227

A drug has 500 mg in the body and a plasma concentration of 10 mg/L. What is its apparent Vd?

A. 5 L
B. 10 L
C. 50 L
D. 500 L

Correct answer: C. 50 L

Explanation: Vd = amount/concentration = 500 mg ÷ 10 mg/L = 50 L.

MCQ 228

A drug with a very small Vd is likely to be:

A. Extensively stored in adipose tissue
B. Primarily confined to plasma
C. Highly distributed into intracellular fluid
D. Completely eliminated

Correct answer: B. Primarily confined to plasma

Explanation: A small Vd indicates that most of the drug remains in the vascular compartment.

MCQ 229

Which drug characteristic tends to increase distribution into adipose tissue?

A. High lipid solubility
B. Permanent ionization
C. Very low lipid solubility
D. Complete plasma confinement

Correct answer: A. High lipid solubility

Explanation: Lipid-soluble drugs may accumulate extensively in adipose tissue.

MCQ 230

The blood-brain barrier generally restricts entry of:

A. Lipid-soluble molecules

B. Small nonionized molecules

C. Many polar molecules

D. Oxygen

Correct answer: C. Many polar molecules

E**xplanation**: The blood-brain barrier limits entry of many polar and ionized substances, while lipid-soluble molecules often cross more readily.

MCQ 231

Drug metabolism is also called:

A. Biotransformation

B. Filtration

C. Diffusion

D. Distribution

Correct answer: A. Biotransformation

Explanation: Drug metabolism refers to enzymatic chemical modification of drugs, usually producing metabolites.

MCQ 232

The major organ responsible for drug metabolism is the:

A. Liver

B. Spleen

C. Pancreas

D. Bone marrow

Correct answer: A. Liver

Explanation: The liver contains numerous enzymes involved in drug metabolism, particularly the cytochrome P450 system.

MCQ 233

Phase I drug metabolism commonly includes:

A. Oxidation

B. Reduction

C. Hydrolysis

D. All of the above

Correct answer: D. All of the above

Explanation: Phase I reactions include oxidation, reduction, and hydrolysis.

MCQ 234

Phase II reactions generally involve:

A. Conjugation

B. Oxidation only

C. Filtration

D. Passive diffusion

Correct answer: A. Conjugation

Explanation: Phase II reactions conjugate drugs or metabolites with endogenous molecules, often increasing water solubility.

MCQ 235

Which enzyme system is particularly important in Phase I metabolism?

A. Cytochrome P450

B. Acetylcholinesterase

C. Na^+/K^+-ATPase

D. DNA polymerase

Correct answer: A. Cytochrome P450

Explanation: Cytochrome P450 enzymes catalyze many oxidative Phase I reactions.

MCQ 236

Enzyme induction generally causes:

A. Reduced metabolism of all drugs

B. Increased metabolism of susceptible drugs

C. Complete inhibition of CYP enzymes

D. Reduced hepatic blood flow only

Correct answer: B. Increased metabolism of susceptible drugs

Explanation: Enzyme inducers increase the activity or expression of metabolic enzymes, potentially reducing concentrations of drugs that are substrates.

MCQ 237

Enzyme inhibition generally causes:

A. Increased metabolism of substrate drugs
B. Reduced metabolism of substrate drugs
C. Increased renal filtration only
D. No change in drug concentrations

Correct answer: B. Reduced metabolism of substrate drugs

Explanation: Enzyme inhibition can decrease drug metabolism and increase plasma concentrations of susceptible substrates.

MCQ 238

A prodrug is:

A. Always pharmacologically inactive after administration
B. Converted in the body to an active drug or active metabolite
C. Always eliminated unchanged
D. A drug that cannot be absorbed

Correct answer: B. Converted in the body to an active drug or active metabolite

Explanation: Prodrugs require metabolic conversion to produce their intended pharmacologic activity.

MCQ 239

Which factor can reduce hepatic drug metabolism?

A. Severe liver dysfunction
B. Increased enzyme activity
C. Enzyme induction
D. Increased hepatic capacity

Correct answer: A. Severe liver dysfunction

Explanation: Significant liver disease can impair metabolism of drugs that depend heavily on hepatic function.

MCQ 240

First-order elimination means:

A. A constant amount is eliminated per unit time

B. A constant fraction is eliminated per unit time

C. Elimination is independent of concentration

D. No drug is eliminated

Correct answer: B. A constant fraction is eliminated per unit time

Explanation: In first-order kinetics, the rate of elimination is proportional to drug concentration, resulting in a constant fraction being removed per unit time.

MCQ 241

Zero-order elimination means:

A. A constant fraction is eliminated per unit time

B. A constant amount is eliminated per unit time

C. Elimination increases exponentially

D. Drug concentration has no relevance

Correct answer: B. A constant amount is eliminated per unit time

Explanation: In zero-order kinetics, elimination pathways are saturated, so a constant amount is eliminated per unit time.

MCQ 242

Which drug is classically associated with zero-order elimination at therapeutic or toxic concentrations?

A. Ethanol

B. Penicillin

C. Gentamicin

D. Atenolol

Correct answer: A. Ethanol

Explanation: Ethanol metabolism follows approximately zero-order kinetics over a clinically relevant concentration range because metabolic pathways become saturated.

MCQ 243

Half-life is the time required for:

A. Complete drug elimination

B. Plasma drug concentration to decrease by 50%

C. Drug concentration to double

D. Absorption to begin

Correct answer: B. Plasma drug concentration to decrease by 50%

Explanation: Half-life is the time required for the amount or concentration of drug to fall by one-half during first-order elimination.

MCQ 244

A drug has a half-life of 4 hours. Approximately what percentage remains after 12 hours?

A. 75%

B. 50%

C. 25%

D. 12.5%

Correct answer: D. 12.5%

Explanation: Twelve hours equals three half-lives. Remaining fraction = 1/2 × 1/2 × 1/2 = 1/8 = 12.5%.

MCQ 245

After approximately how many half-lives is more than 95% of a first-order drug eliminated?

A. 1

B. 2

C. 3

D. 5

Correct answer: D. 5

Explanation: After about five half-lives, approximately 97% of a drug has been eliminated.

MCQ 246

The half-life of a drug is influenced by:

A. Clearance

B. Volume of distribution

C. Both A and B

D. Neither A nor B

Correct answer: C. Both A and B

Explanation: For first-order elimination, $t_{1/2} = 0.693 \times Vd / CL$.

MCQ 247

If clearance decreases while Vd remains constant, the half-life will:

A. Decrease

B. Increase

C. Remain unchanged

D. Become zero

Correct answer: B. Increase

Explanation: Since half-life is inversely related to clearance, reduced clearance prolongs half-life.

MCQ 248

Clearance is best defined as:

A. The amount of drug absorbed

B. The volume of plasma cleared of drug per unit time

C. The total amount of drug administered

D. The amount of drug bound to protein

Correct answer: B. The volume of plasma cleared of drug per unit time

Explanation: Clearance represents the efficiency of drug elimination and is expressed as volume/time.

MCQ 249

Total body clearance is approximately the sum of:

A. Renal and hepatic clearance only

B. All relevant organ clearances

C. Absorption and distribution

D. Bioavailability and Vd

Correct answer: B. All relevant organ clearances

Explanation: Total clearance is the sum of clearance by the kidneys, liver, and other organs capable of eliminating the drug.

MCQ 250

A drug has a plasma concentration of 5 mg/L and is eliminated at 25 mg/hour. What is its clearance?

A. 2 L/hour

B. 5 L/hour

C. 10 L/hour

D. 125 L/hour

Correct answer: B. 5 L/hour

Explanation: Clearance = elimination rate ÷ concentration = 25 mg/hour ÷ 5 mg/L = 5 L/hour.

MCQ 251

Renal clearance depends on:

A. Glomerular filtration

B. Tubular secretion

C. Tubular reabsorption

D. All of the above

Correct answer: D. All of the above

Explanation: Renal drug elimination is determined by filtration, secretion, and reabsorption.

MCQ 252

Only the following fraction of a drug is readily filtered through the glomerulus:

A. Protein-bound drug

B. Unbound drug

C. Drug stored in tissue

D. Drug inside red blood cells only

Correct answer: B. Unbound drug

Explanation: Large protein-bound drug complexes generally do not pass readily through the glomerular filtration barrier.

MCQ 253

Active tubular secretion occurs primarily in the:

A. Proximal tubule

B. Loop of Henle only

C. Collecting duct only

D. Glomerulus

Correct answer: A. Proximal tubule

Explanation: Transport systems in the proximal tubule actively secrete various organic acids and bases into tubular fluid.

MCQ 254

Tubular reabsorption generally:

A. Promotes drug elimination
B. Returns drug from tubular fluid to blood
C. Occurs only by active transport
D. Prevents all renal elimination

Correct answer: B. Returns drug from tubular fluid to blood

Explanation: Reabsorption transfers drug from tubular fluid back into the systemic circulation, potentially reducing renal elimination.

MCQ 255

Which property favors passive tubular reabsorption?

A. Lipid solubility
B. Permanent ionization
C. High polarity
D. Strong water solubility

Correct answer: A. Lipid solubility

Explanation: Lipid-soluble, nonionized drugs can passively diffuse across tubular membranes and may be reabsorbed.

MCQ 256

Alkalinization of urine tends to increase the renal elimination of:

A. Weak acids
B. Weak bases
C. Neutral compounds only
D. All drugs equally

Correct answer: A. Weak acids

Explanation: Alkaline urine increases ionization of weak acids, reducing their tubular reabsorption and increasing excretion.

MCQ 257

Acidification of urine tends to increase elimination of:

A. Weak acids
B. Weak bases
C. Neutral drugs
D. Lipid-soluble neutral molecules

Correct answer: B. Weak bases

Explanation: Acidic urine increases ionization of weak bases, reducing reabsorption and promoting urinary excretion.

MCQ 258

Creatinine clearance is commonly used clinically as an estimate of:

A. Hepatic clearance
B. Glomerular filtration rate
C. Drug absorption
D. Drug bioavailability

Correct answer: B. Glomerular filtration rate

Explanation: Creatinine clearance provides an estimate of renal filtration function and is useful when adjusting doses of renally eliminated drugs.

MCQ 259

A drug eliminated primarily by the kidneys may require dose adjustment in:

A. Renal impairment
B. Hyperthyroidism only
C. Increased gastric acidity only
D. Skin disease

Correct answer: A. Renal impairment

Explanation: Reduced renal function can decrease clearance and cause accumulation of renally eliminated drugs.

MCQ 260

Which organ is the major route for elimination of many water-soluble drugs?

A. Kidney

C. Spleen

B. Skin

D. Bone

Correct answer: A. Kidney

Explanation: The kidneys eliminate many drugs and metabolites through urine.

MCQ 261

A loading dose is primarily used to:

A. Maintain a stable concentration indefinitely
B. Rapidly achieve a desired therapeutic concentration
C. Reduce drug absorption
D. Increase renal elimination

Correct answer: B. Rapidly achieve a desired therapeutic concentration

Explanation: A loading dose is designed to achieve the target plasma concentration more rapidly than repeated maintenance doses alone.

MCQ 262

The loading dose is particularly influenced by:

A. Volume of distribution
B. Clearance only
C. Urine pH only
D. Gastric emptying only

Correct answer: A. Volume of distribution

Explanation: A simplified loading-dose equation is Loading dose = target concentration × Vd / F.

MCQ 263

The maintenance dose is primarily determined by:

A. Clearance
B. Hair color
C. Volume of the stomach
D. Drug taste

Correct answer: A. Clearance

Explanation: Maintenance dosing is designed to replace the amount of drug eliminated and therefore depends strongly on clearance.

MCQ 264

A patient requires a target plasma concentration of 10 mg/L. If Vd is 50 L and bioavailability is 100%, the approximate loading dose is:

A. 50 mg
B. 100 mg
C. 500 mg
D. 5,000 mg

Correct answer: C. 500 mg

Explanation: Loading dose = target concentration × Vd / F = 10 × 50 / 1 = 500 mg.

MCQ 265

If oral bioavailability is 50%, compared with an equivalent IV dose, the oral dose required to achieve the same systemic exposure is generally:

A. Half
B. The same
C. Approximately twice as large
D. Ten times larger in all cases

Correct answer: C. Approximately twice as large

Explanation: If F = 0.5, approximately twice the oral dose is required to provide the same systemic amount as an equivalent IV dose, assuming linear kinetics.

MCQ 266

Steady-state concentration during repeated dosing is reached when:

A. Absorption stops
B. Rate of drug administration equals rate of elimination
C. All drug is protein bound
D. The drug is completely metabolized
Correct answer: B. Rate of drug administration equals rate of elimination

Explanation: At steady state, the average rate of drug input equals the average rate of drug elimination.

MCQ 267

Approximately what percentage of steady state is reached after one half-life?

A. 25%
B. 50%
C. 75%
D. 100%

Correct answer: B. 50%

Explanation: After one half-life, approximately 50% of the eventual steady-state concentration is achieved.

MCQ 268

Approximately what percentage of steady state is reached after four half-lives?

A. 50%
B. 75%
C. 94%
D. 100%

Correct answer: C. 94%

Explanation: After four half-lives, approximately 94% of steady state has been reached.

MCQ 269

Increasing the dose of a linearly eliminated drug generally causes:

A. A proportional increase in plasma concentration
B. No change in concentration
C. A decrease in concentration
D. Complete elimination

Correct answer: A. A proportional increase in plasma concentration

Explanation: In linear pharmacokinetics, dose and concentration increase proportionally within the relevant range.

MCQ 270

Saturable pharmacokinetics may occur when:

A. Metabolic enzymes become saturated
B. Drug concentration is always zero
C. There is no drug absorption
D. The drug is administered intravenously

Correct answer: A. Metabolic enzymes become saturated

Explanation: Saturation of enzymes or transport systems can cause nonlinear pharmacokinetics.

MCQ 271

In nonlinear pharmacokinetics:

A. Dose and plasma concentration may not be proportional
B. Half-life is always constant
C. Clearance is always constant
D. Elimination is always first-order

Correct answer: A. Dose and plasma concentration may not be proportional

Explanation: Saturation can cause disproportionate changes in concentration when the dose is changed.

MCQ 272

Which is an important consequence of nonlinear pharmacokinetics?

A. Small dose increases may cause disproportionately large increases in concentration

B. Dose adjustments are always unnecessary

C. Toxicity is impossible

D. Plasma concentration never changes

Correct answer: A. Small dose increases may cause disproportionately large increases in concentration

Explanation: Once an elimination pathway becomes saturated, additional doses may produce disproportionately high drug concentrations.

MCQ 273

Therapeutic drug monitoring is particularly useful for drugs with:

A. Wide therapeutic indices only

B. Narrow therapeutic indices

C. No systemic absorption

D. No pharmacologic effects

Correct answer: B. Narrow therapeutic indices

Explanation: Drugs with a narrow therapeutic index have a relatively small margin between effective and toxic concentrations.

MCQ 274

Which is an important purpose of therapeutic drug monitoring?

A. To measure drug concentration when concentration-response relationships are clinically useful

B. To determine patient blood type

C. To diagnose all infections

D. To replace clinical assessment

Correct answer: A. To measure drug concentration when concentration-response relationships are clinically useful

Explanation: Drug levels can help optimize therapy for selected medications, particularly those with narrow therapeutic ranges.

MCQ 275

A trough concentration is generally measured:

A. Immediately after a dose
B. Just before the next dose
C. During drug absorption only
D. Before the first dose in every case

Correct answer: B. Just before the next dose

Explanation: A trough is the lowest concentration during a dosing interval and is typically measured immediately before the next dose.

MCQ 276

A peak concentration is generally:

A. The lowest concentration during the dosing interval
B. The highest concentration during the dosing interval
C. Always measured before administration
D. Unrelated to dosing

Correct answer: B. The highest concentration during the dosing interval

Explanation: Peak concentration represents the maximum measured drug concentration after administration, depending on the drug and route.

MCQ 277

Which factor can increase the half-life of a drug?

A. Increased clearance
B. Decreased volume of distribution
C. Decreased clearance
D. Increased renal elimination

Correct answer: C. Decreased clearance

Explanation: Reduced clearance slows elimination and therefore prolongs half-life.

MCQ 278

If the Vd of a drug doubles while clearance remains unchanged, the half-life will approximately:

A. Be halved
B. Double
C. Remain unchanged
D. Become zero

Correct answer: B. Double

Explanation: Since t½ is proportional to Vd when clearance is constant, doubling Vd approximately doubles the half-life.

MCQ 279

A drug has a Vd of 40 L and a clearance of 5 L/hour. Its approximate half-life is:

A. 0.55 hours
B. 2.8 hours
C. 5.5 hours
D. 40 hours

Correct answer: C. 5.5 hours

Explanation: t½ = 0.693 × Vd / CL = 0.693 × 40 / 5 ≈ 5.5 hours.

MCQ 280

Which change would most likely increase plasma concentration of a drug eliminated by hepatic metabolism?

A. Increased hepatic clearance
B. Decreased hepatic clearance
C. Increased renal clearance
D. Increased drug elimination

Correct answer: B. Decreased hepatic clearance

Explanation: Reduced clearance causes slower elimination and therefore tends to increase plasma drug concentration.

MCQ 281

A drug has an elimination half-life of 6 hours. Approximately how much remains after 18 hours?

A. 75%
B. 50%
C. 25%
D. 12.5%

Correct answer: D. 12.5%

Explanation: Eighteen hours represents three half-lives: 100% → 50% → 25% → 12.5%.

MCQ 282

A drug's plasma concentration falls from 80 mg/L to 40 mg/L in 5 hours. If first-order kinetics apply, the half-life is:

A. 2.5 hours
B. 5 hours
C. 10 hours
D. 40 hours

Correct answer: B. 5 hours

Explanation: The concentration decreased by 50% in 5 hours, so the half-life is 5 hours.

MCQ 283

If a drug's clearance doubles and its dosing rate remains unchanged, its average steady-state concentration will approximately:

A. Double
B. Decrease by half
C. Remain unchanged
D. Increase fourfold

Correct answer: B. Decrease by half

Explanation: For linear kinetics, average steady-state concentration is proportional to dosing rate divided by clearance.

MCQ 284

If the maintenance dosing rate is doubled while clearance remains constant, the average steady-state concentration will approximately:

A. Decrease by half

B. Remain unchanged

C. Double

D. Increase tenfold

Correct answer: C. Double

Explanation: In linear pharmacokinetics, doubling the dosing rate approximately doubles the average steady-state concentration.

MCQ 285

Which factor can alter oral drug absorption?

A. Gastric emptying

B. Intestinal motility

C. Presence of food

D. All of the above

Correct answer: D. All of the above

Explanation: Gastrointestinal physiology and food can influence the rate and sometimes the extent of drug absorption.

MCQ 286

Enterohepatic recirculation can:

A. Shorten drug exposure in all cases

B. Prolong the presence of some drugs in the body

C. Prevent hepatic metabolism

D. Eliminate the need for renal excretion

Correct answer: B. Prolong the presence of some drugs in the body

Explanation: Some drugs or metabolites are excreted into bile, enter the intestine, and may be reabsorbed, prolonging exposure.

MCQ 287

Which organ is particularly important for biliary drug excretion?

A. Liver

B. Thyroid

C. Pancreas

D. Bone marrow

Correct answer: A. Liver

Explanation: Hepatocytes can transport drugs and metabolites into bile, which then enters the gastrointestinal tract.

MCQ 288

Drug elimination through the lungs is particularly important for:

A. Volatile substances

B. Large protein-bound molecules

C. Insoluble tablets

D. Highly polar proteins

Correct answer: A. Volatile substances

Explanation: Volatile compounds, such as some anesthetic agents, can be eliminated through the lungs.

MCQ 289

Which pharmacokinetic parameter is most directly related to the extent of drug distribution?

A. Volume of distribution

B. Clearance

C. Bioavailability

D. Renal secretion

Correct answer: A. Volume of distribution

Explanation: Vd provides an estimate of the apparent extent to which a drug distributes outside the plasma.

MCQ 290

A drug with extensive tissue binding is likely to have:

A. A relatively large Vd
B. A very small Vd in all cases
C. No tissue distribution
D. 100% renal clearance

Correct answer: A. A relatively large Vd

Explanation: Extensive tissue binding can lower plasma concentration relative to the total amount in the body, producing a large apparent Vd.

MCQ 291

Which condition can increase the free fraction of a highly protein-bound drug?

A. Increased plasma albumin
B. Reduced plasma albumin
C. Increased binding affinity
D. Increased protein concentration

Correct answer: B. Reduced plasma albumin

Explanation: Reduced albumin concentration can decrease available binding sites and increase the unbound fraction of some drugs.

MCQ 292

A highly protein-bound drug is displaced from albumin by another drug. The immediate effect may be:

A. Decreased free drug concentration
B. Increased free drug concentration
C. Complete elimination
D. Complete absorption

Correct answer: B. Increased free drug concentration

Explanation: Displacement from protein-binding sites can transiently increase the free fraction, although the clinical effect depends on subsequent distribution and clearance.

MCQ 293

Which statement about renal drug elimination is correct?

A. Protein-bound drug is freely filtered

B. Tubular secretion can contribute to elimination

C. Reabsorption always increases elimination

D. Filtration is the only renal mechanism

Correct answer: B. Tubular secretion can contribute to elimination

Explanation: Renal elimination involves filtration, active secretion, and reabsorption.

MCQ 294

A drug is eliminated by glomerular filtration and active tubular secretion, with minimal reabsorption. Its renal clearance may be:

A. Greater than the filtration clearance alone

B. Zero

C. Always equal to bioavailability

D. Less than zero

Correct answer: A. Greater than the filtration clearance alone

Explanation: Active tubular secretion adds drug to the tubular fluid and can increase renal clearance beyond filtration alone.

MCQ 295

Which statement best describes pharmacokinetic drug interactions?

A. One drug changes the absorption, distribution, metabolism, or excretion of another drug

B. One drug always blocks the receptor of another

C. They occur only at the receptor

D. They cannot change plasma drug concentrations

Correct answer: A. One drug changes the absorption, distribution, metabolism, or excretion of another drug

Explanation: Pharmacokinetic interactions alter drug concentrations by affecting ADME processes.

MCQ 296

An enzyme inhibitor is added to a patient taking a drug metabolized by that enzyme. What is the most likely initial effect?

A. Increased metabolism of the drug

B. Decreased plasma concentration

C. Reduced metabolism and potentially increased plasma concentration

D. Complete elimination of the drug

Correct answer: C. Reduced metabolism and potentially increased plasma concentration

Explanation: Enzyme inhibition can decrease metabolic clearance and increase systemic exposure to the substrate drug.

MCQ 297

A patient with severe renal impairment receives a drug that is primarily eliminated unchanged by the kidneys. Which outcome is most likely?

A. Increased drug clearance

B. Decreased half-life

C. Drug accumulation

D. Increased renal excretion

Correct answer: C. Drug accumulation

Explanation: Reduced renal clearance can increase plasma concentrations and prolong the drug's half-life, leading to accumulation.

MCQ 298

A patient receives repeated doses of a drug with first-order elimination. If the dosing interval is shortened without changing the dose, the average drug concentration will generally:

A. Increase

B. Decrease

C. Become zero

D. Remain exactly unchanged

Correct answer: A. Increase

Explanation: Shortening the dosing interval increases the total dosing rate, which generally increases the average steady-state concentration when clearance is unchanged.

MCQ 299

A drug has a bioavailability of 0.8. Which oral dose would provide approximately the same systemic amount as 80 mg administered intravenously?

A. 40 mg

B. 64 mg

C. 80 mg

D. 100 mg

Correct answer: D. 100 mg

Explanation: Oral dose × F = IV dose. Therefore, oral dose = 80 ÷ 0.8 = 100 mg.

MCQ 300

Which statement best summarizes the relationship among absorption, distribution, metabolism, and excretion?

A. They are unrelated processes

B. They collectively determine the concentration and duration of drug exposure in the body

C. Only metabolism determines drug concentration

D. Only absorption determines drug action

Correct answer: B. They collectively determine the concentration and duration of drug exposure in the body

Explanation: Pharmacokinetics integrates absorption, distribution, metabolism, and excretion to determine drug concentrations over time and therefore strongly influences drug exposure.

References

- Brunton, L. L., Hilal-Dandan, R., & Knollmann, B. C., eds. Goodman & Gilman's The Pharmacological Basis of Therapeutics. McGraw Hill.
- Katzung, B. G., & Vanderah, T. W. Basic & Clinical Pharmacology. McGraw Hill.
- Ritter, J. M., Flower, R. J., Henderson, G., Loke, Y. K., MacEwan, D., & Rang, H. P. Rang & Dale's Pharmacology. Elsevier.
- Whalen, K. Lippincott Illustrated Reviews: Pharmacology. Wolters Kluwer.
- Katzung, B. G. Trevor's Basic & Clinical Pharmacology Review. McGraw Hill.
- Rowland, M., & Tozer, T. N. Clinical Pharmacokinetics and Pharmacodynamics: Concepts and Applications. Wolters Kluwer.
- Shargel, L., Wu-Pong, S., & Yu, A. B. C. Applied Biopharmaceutics & Pharmacokinetics. McGraw Hill.
- Derendorf, H., & Schmidt, S. Rowland and Tozer's Clinical Pharmacokinetics and Pharmacodynamics: Concepts and Applications. Wolters Kluwer.